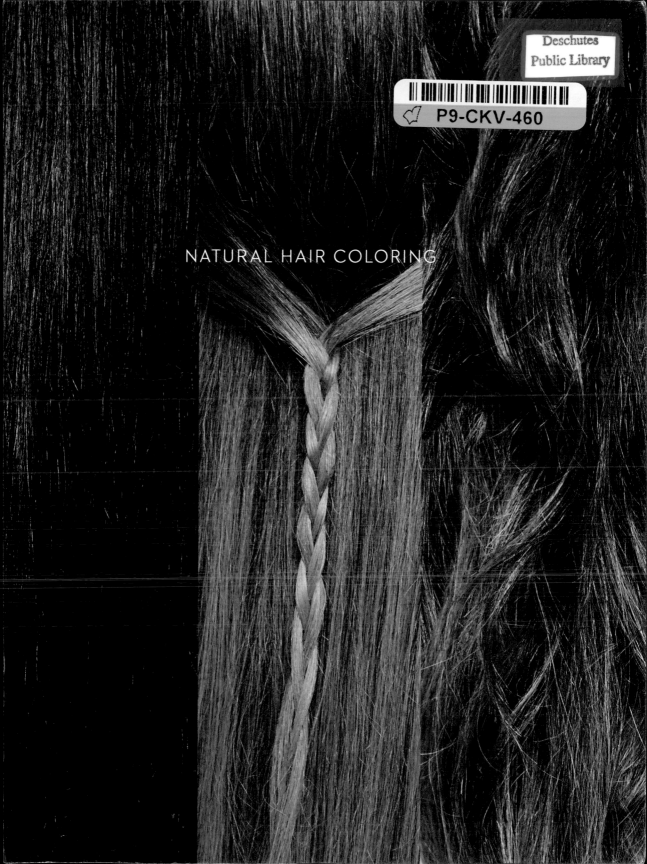

NATURAL HAIR COLORING

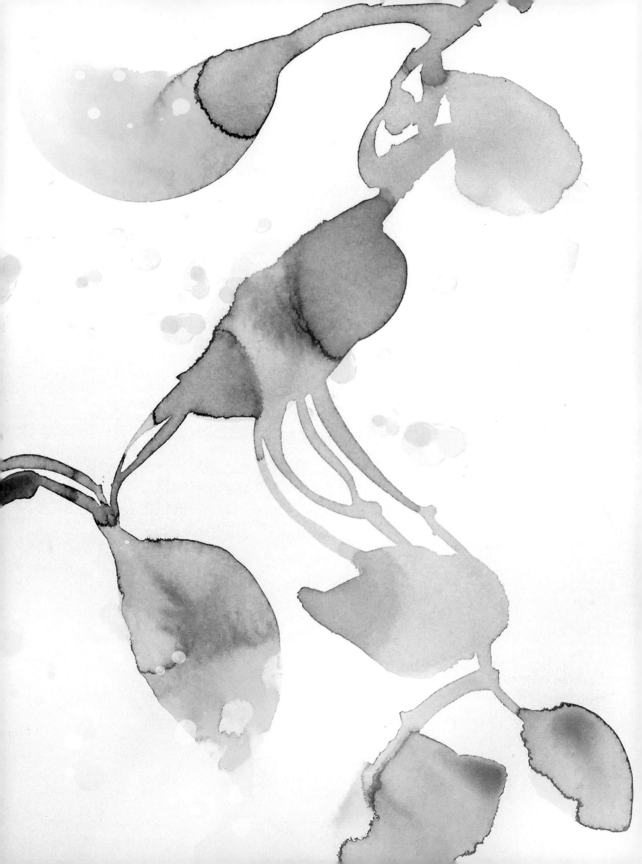

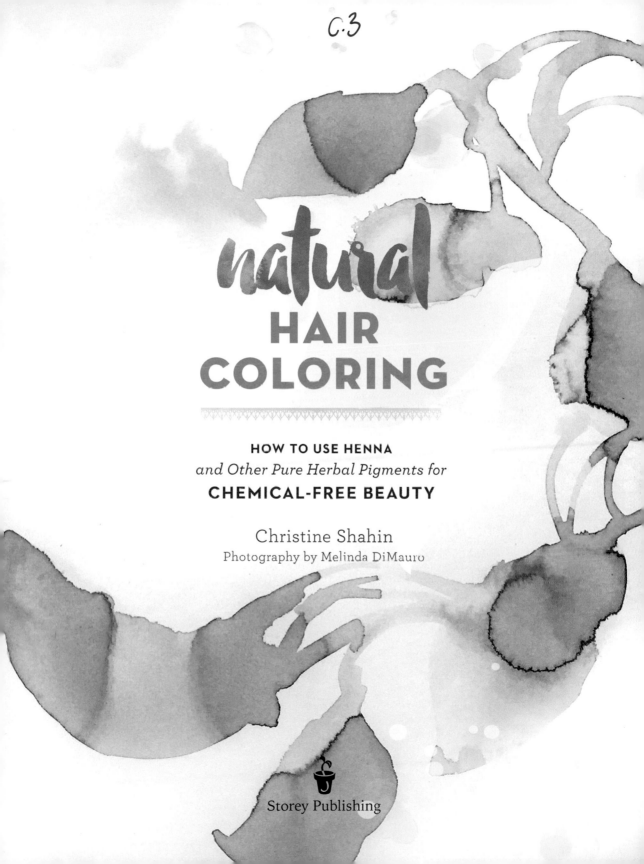

C.3

natural HAIR COLORING

HOW TO USE HENNA
and Other Pure Herbal Pigments for
CHEMICAL-FREE BEAUTY

Christine Shahin

Photography by Melinda DiMauro

Storey Publishing

The mission of Storey Publishing is to serve our customers by publishing practical information that encourages personal independence in harmony with the environment.

Edited by Deborah Balmuth and Sarah Guare
Art direction and book design by
    Alethea Morrison
Indexed by Christine R. Lindemer, Boston Road
    Communications

Cover and interior photography by
    © Melinda DiMauro, except for:
    © Andreas Kuehn/Getty Images, 31; © Diamond
    Sky Images/Getty Images, 29; © 2014 Erin
    Covey Creative, back cover (author), 17;
    © Fancy Photography/Veer.com, 168; © 2011
    Gamma-Keystone/Getty Images, 144 (left);
    © Hulton Archive/Getty Images, 144 (right);
    © 2014 John Bulmer/Getty Images, 145;
    © JPM/Getty Images, 26; Mars Vilaubi, 76,
    105, 152, 161, 163; © Matthieu Paley/Getty
    Images, 40; © Michele Mossop/Getty Images,
    63; Moses Harris color wheel/Wikimedia
    Commons, 98

Illustrations © Marta Spendowska,
    except page 35 © Jane Kim

Be sure to follow instructions as given and adhere to all recommended safety guidelines. Follow the instructions for doing a patch test on page 109 and consult a physician if any adverse reaction occurs. This publication is not intended to take the place of personalized medical counseling, diagnosis, and treatment from a trained health professional.

The information in this book is true and complete to the best of our knowledge. All recommendations are made without guarantee on the part of the author or Storey Publishing. The author and publisher disclaim any liability in connection with the use of this information.

Storey books are available for special premium and promotional uses and for customized editions. For further information, please call 1-800-793-9396.

Storey Publishing
210 MASS MoCA Way
North Adams, MA 01247
www.storey.com

Printed in China by Reliance Printing (SZ)
Co., Ltd.
10 9 8 7 6 5 4 3 2 1

Library of Congress Cataloging-in-Publication Data

Names: Shahin, Christine, author.
    Title: Natural hair coloring : how to use henna and other pure herbal pigments for chemical-free beauty / Christine Shahin.
    Description: North Adams, MA : Storey Publishing, [2016]
    Identifiers: LCCN 2015044814| ISBN 9781612125985 (pbk. : alk. paper) | ISBN 9781612125992 (ebook)
    Subjects: LCSH: Hair—Dyeing and bleaching. | Hair dyes. | Plant pigments.
    Classification: LCC TT973 .S53 2016 | DDC 646.7/24—dc23
    LC record available at http://lccn.loc.gov/2015044814

DEDICATION

In memory of Terry Darling, L.C.
— thank you for the keys

Thank you, Creator, for my life and all experiences.
I am grateful too for any beneficent results that may
come from it for others.

I dedicate this book to Planet Earth. May we know,
love, and abide by your natural laws as we mature in
our interstellar experience, affirming our rightful place
in the one song known as Universe.

To Astarte, goddess of beauty and love with a little
war on the side, thank you for your example of how to
integrate these seemingly opposite models.

To Henna, Indigo, Cassia, and Amla, thank you for
your gifts of healing and color and for our relationship.

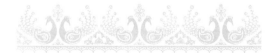

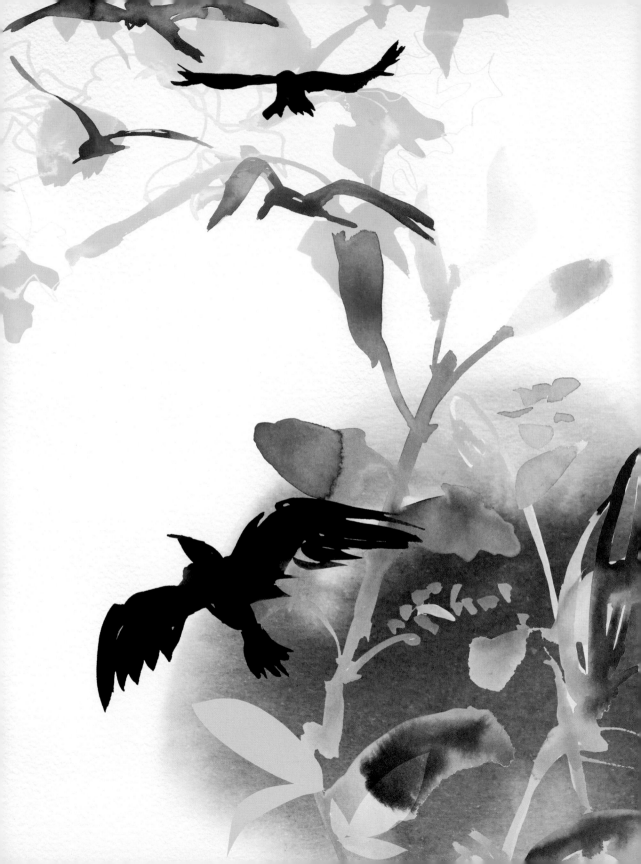

Beauty is not a need but an ecstasy.

It is not a mouth thirsting
nor an empty hand stretched forth,
But rather a heart enflamed and a soul enchanted.

It is not the image you would see
nor the song you would hear,
But rather an image you see though you close your
eyes and a song you hear though you shut your ears.

It is not the sap within the furrowed bark,
nor a wing attached to a claw,
But rather a garden for ever in bloom and a flock of
angels for ever in flight.

People of Orphalese,
beauty is life when life unveils her holy face.
But you are life and you are the veil.

Beauty is eternity gazing at itself in a mirror.
But you are eternity and you are the mirror.

KHALIL GIBRAN, FROM *THE PROPHET*

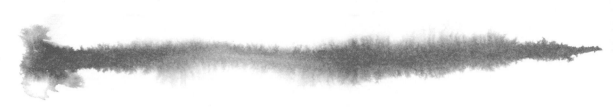

CONTENTS

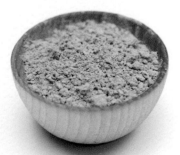
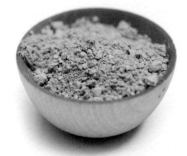
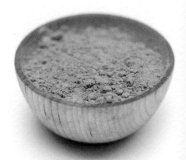

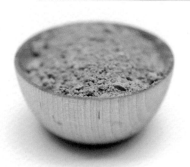

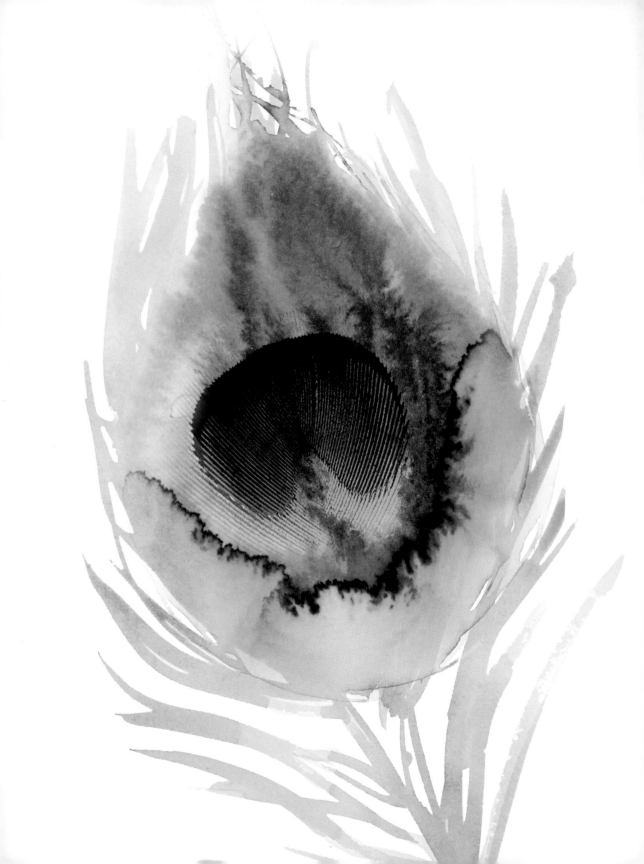

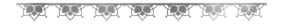

FOREWORD

I fell in love with henna when I first discovered it in my early teens and became an official "mudhead." I love the rich red highlights it creates in my dark brown hair, and I have used it regularly, almost religiously, for many years.

As invariably happens when I discover something I love, I want to share it with others. Soon I was convincing everyone I could to try henna! There was almost always a henna session after the herb classes I offered, and I'd have henna parties at my large herbal conferences, where I would henna 20 to 30 people at a time. I even took henna with me on my "Plant Lovers Journeys." My travel companions and I once used it around a campfire in the jungles of Belize, once on a riverbank in the far outback of Patagonia, several times in the courtyard of an Italian villa in Tuscany, and once in a provincial farmhouse in a small French village. We'd sit around in the warm sun, sipping tea and talking of those things that mattered most in life until the henna had done its magic. It was such fun to watch people rinse out the green-hued paste and discover vibrant shades of red, copper, and brown, along with rich golden highlights.

But it was more than just the colorful highlights and the conditioning effect that seemed to draw people to henna; an actual transformation happened during the mudding process, an enchantment that made people feel better. This is what I love best about henna — it not only makes people's hair light up, but it also seems to make them glow from within.

Recently, I was sent something fabulous in the mail: a copy of this book. Absolutely the best book on natural hair care and coloring I've ever come across, it captures both the magic and the art of natural hair care. Christine is a coloring maestro who has had years of experience using natural colorants, and she shares her knowledge generously and warmly. Included in her wonderfully comprehensive book are all of the reasons for coloring (or not coloring) your hair with natural colorants, instructions on how to mix and apply muds, fabulous color formulations, recipes for shampoos and conditioners, and information on what *not* to do. Written with such beauty and sensitivity and accented with the loveliest quotes, *Natural Hair Coloring* is a pleasure to read.

Christine is adept at blending henna with other supportive herbs to "tone down" the bright red and orange hues that sometimes result from henna, and she has developed some particularly unique combinations for conditioning challenging hair. Thank you, Christine, for your beautiful, radiant book, and for sharing your knowledge and experience with such beauty and wisdom. You've made it all so much fun.

"What we do with our hair has had powerful symbolic and emotional effects in every culture for thousands of years," says Christine . . . may our stories continue!

In gratitude,
ROSEMARY GLADSTAR
Best-selling author of *Rosemary Gladstar's Medicinal Herbs: A Beginner's Guide*

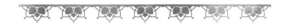

PREFACE

The appearance of things changes
according to the emotions, and thus we
see magic and beauty in them, while the
magic and beauty are really in ourselves.

KHALIL GIBRAN

I am excited to be writing this book about coloring hair with natural herbal colorants after many years of practice! Here I sit thinking about what to share with you regarding my natural beauty journey and how it's evolved into the current manifestation of this book. It's a story that started a long time ago, but don't they all?

My paternal grandparents emigrated from Lebanon during the Great Depression. My father, born Khalil, was one of seven children. His mother died when he was 12 years old, and per her deathbed wish, my father became an Antiochian Orthodox Christian priest. One of my most influential experiences growing up was summer church camp in the midst of the Allegheny Mountains. Sunrise services and evening vespers surrounded by flora and fauna connected me spiritually to the environment.

My mother was born to Lebanese American parents near Beirut. She grew up there until the age of 16, when she left her two sisters, uncle, and aunt to come live with her father in Elmira, New York. My formative years were strongly influenced by Arabic Christian culture within an American culture, making me "bicultural," as our daughter Shadia says.

Growing up, I was interested in fashion and had many good examples of beauty. Beauty is important in both my cultures, as a sign of self-care, self-respect, and self-expression. Lebanese women across the world tend to be very fashion-conscious, as were my mother and her sisters, including the eldest, Esther, a store model I aspired to emulate. My mother Jeanine, a petite woman who always received

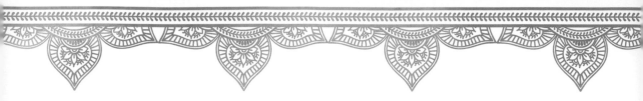

compliments and wore no makeup, except for some lipstick on occasion, would put her thick, butt-length black hair in a top chignon; her style was simple elegance.

Though I never witnessed my mother in front of a mirror applying makeup (she did practice daily skin care and continues to do so to this day), using makeup came quite instinctively to me. I purchased my first eye pencil and foundation at age 13. As Mama and I grew together, there were rare occasions when she would ask me to do her makeup. This same request spontaneously came from friends and classmates for special occasions, though I never considered beauty as a career. People always inquired of my ethnicity, and I always seemed to be fighting it, trying to look more mainstream by ironing my hair, bleaching facial hair, and having electrolysis on my eyebrows starting at age 12.

I began turning more toward a natural expression of beauty as I bloomed into a "flower child." I was 16 when Martin Luther King Jr. and Bobby Kennedy were assassinated. With the focus on society's weightier issues of racial equality, women's rights, environmental degradation, and war, many people were choosing to be less primped, forgoing makeup and elaborate hairstyles. All of these influences impacted my personal understanding of, connection with, and approach to beauty.

In our mid-twenties, my husband, Steven, and I moved to the foothills of the Adirondack Mountains, where we gardened and raised our six children "naturally." Folklore and herbal remedies were our immediate response to health needs. We chose this approach because these remedies are food-based. With this knowledge, we are self-empowered and self-sustaining, as many healing plants can be grown at home and stored for use when needed. We also liked that these remedies have less of an environmental impact than conventional treatments, especially when organically grown, because the unused or waste materials are more readily returned to nature, from whence they came. Recognizing that beauty products, too, could be much safer for the environment, I decided to go to cosmetology school with the intention of one day creating an all-natural beauty salon.

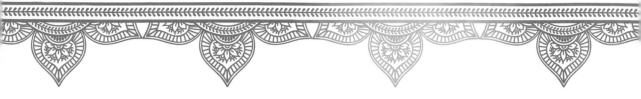

That day started to unfold when, after decades of eco-activism, I took a position at a premier health store in the city of Syracuse seeking a licensed cosmetologist for their cutting-edge health and beauty department. One day my employer asked why I didn't color my hair using the "natural" hair colors she carried so that I would have experience with these products and could be a guide for customers. I decided to color my hair with a henna line she carried. Results were good! The gray was gone, and my hair and color looked natural. Thus began my herbal colorant journey.

I started my eco-salon, Faces of Astarte, in 2006, in a small booth in an old mill that had been turned into an artisan vendors mall. There I consulted on the best practices for maintaining healthy, natural hair and skin and sold products. In a short time, the booth morphed into an elegant eco-salon and spa in the same area on the Mohawk River, nestled between ridges. I still offer consultations on the best practices for healthy, natural hair and skin, but Faces of Astarte is now a full-service salon with facial spa services. I provide cleaner, safer, less toxic versions of chemical colors and perms, though my main focus is on coloring hair with pure herbal pigments and doing noninvasive face-lift facials.

WHAT IS AN ECO-SALON?

There is no standard definition of what an "eco-salon" is, though you will see many salons claiming to be one. My personal expression of what an eco-salon looks like differs from what you will find in mainstream versions. Typically, though, eco-salons use beauty products that are cleaner, safer, and less toxic than those found in standard salons. The National Association for Eco-Friendly Salons & Spas (NAEFSS) is a wonderful organization and network for salons and spas that want to step up to sustainability. The organization also offers a rigorous certification process for its members, so consumers are assured that the salon/spa is what it claims to be. This process benefits both the service provider and the consumer.

Repeatedly, patrons affirm their appreciation for the peaceful ambience of Faces of Astarte — its clean and earthy smells, eclectic décor, relaxed pace, soothing music, and spaciousness help foster authentic conversations that pave the way for strangers to become friends. It is interesting that several of my clients have commented to me that my salon is true to the word's origins: the word *salon* first appeared in 1664 in France and became a fashionable term for "an important place for the exchange of cutting-edge thoughts." Often, visitors to the area will walk in because they are drawn by the character and feel of the outside and window display only to be surprised to find a salon — and proceed to make an appointment!

In this book, I share my personal experience with the four herbs I use daily in Faces of Astarte Salon: henna, indigo, amla, and cassia obovata. Initially, people paid me, albeit lower rates than now, to experiment on their willing heads! In time, I gained a basic knowledge that I could faithfully apply to my clients. I am excited to share with you how to use these herbal colorants to your benefit.

When I discovered henna and the other herbal colorants, something resonated deeply inside me; I am still that little girl who never grew out of playing in the mud or daring to follow the beat of her own drum. I have taken traditional and current wisdom and tested it for myself, not because I wanted to reinvent the wheel but because I wanted to know firsthand how everything worked, from color combinations to timing to mixing pigments. I encourage you to do the same — don't just take my word for it. Get exploratory, get playful, and get into the herbal muds!

This book shares many of the discoveries that have emerged from my personal quest to live fully in this time and live in harmony with nature's laws as much as possible. In no way is this an end to experimenting with these colorants — the journey continues!

May the contents of these pages — gained from years of living in Eastern- and Western-infused cultures, imbibing others' herbal wisdom, exploring with trial and error, and tapping into my own instincts — enhance your ability to live your values.

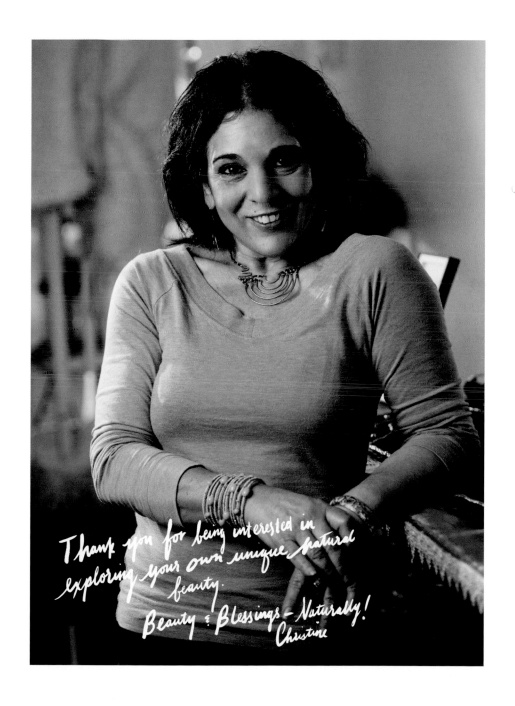

Thank you for being interested in exploring your own unique, natural beauty.

Beauty & Blessings — Naturally!
Christine

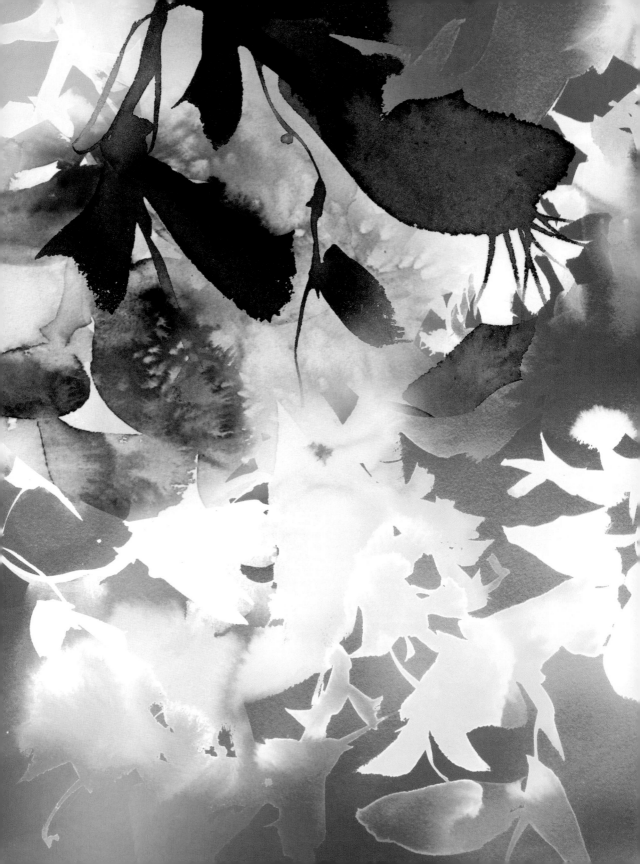

WELLNESS BEAUTY AND SAGE-ING

Nobody grows old merely by living a number of years. We grow old by deserting our ideals. Years may wrinkle the skin, but to give up enthusiasm wrinkles the soul.

SAMUEL ULLMAN

The beauty spoken of here in these pages is your own. It is the natural beauty of self-discovery and diversity, your unique expression of genetics, culture, and style.

Beauty customs (common practices being hair and skin care and makeup) have continued to evolve in all cultures for thousands of years. They often began as holistic practices that benefited the health of the individual as well as the environment. Over time, health was separated more and more from beauty, until society began to view beauty issues through a medical lens that turned them into problems that need to be "fixed." I believe our society's story has reached a point where we're ready to embrace another beauty, what I call wellness beauty.

Some will automatically assume wellness beauty is synonymous with diet and supplementation, and while these tools can be helpful, if we view them as a panacea, we lose sight of the body's miraculous and innate ability to function without our worrying about it. I use the term *wellness beauty* to indicate an integrated approach of mind, body, and spirit that recognizes that each aspect of the self needs its particular nourishment, food, or "supplementation" — whether it's sunshine, movement, or meditation.

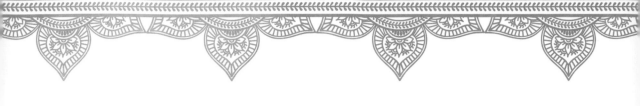

The pure herbal colorants described in this book are plants that have been used for centuries for healing, and some have been used just as long for color. Coming from the earth, they grow in various geographies and climates. The very elements of air, earth, and water, along with the light of the sun, moon, and stars, all combine to create the conditions that impact these plants' ability to not only heal but also serve cosmetic purposes. In this way, herbal colorants connect us more deeply with the earth and our universe and can be a part of a wellness beauty lifestyle.

As we embrace wellness beauty, so too may we embody conscious aging, known also as "sage-ing." Sage-ing is a part of a broader movement that, according to Sage-ing International (sage-ing.org), "offers a vision of aging as a time of life characterized not by diminishment and decline, but by growth, contribution, and fulfillment." The organization strives to "change the paradigm in our culture from age-ing to sage-ing." We grow older and sage rather than decline and age.

Regardless of our current age, we all grow older from the time we are born, so this is not a message just for those older than 50, but an ongoing conversation for people at every stage or "season" of life. Everything experiences seasons. There are general planetary seasons of spring, summer, autumn, and winter as well as perpetual shifts from drought to flood to bountiful harvest within those cycles. We experience seasons as we progress from infant to elder, and we each have personal seasons within these when we are insecure/confident, unemployed/productive, depressed/shining. These fluctuating influences touch all aspects of our lives — physically, emotionally, spiritually — and change the way we view beauty, as our self-expressive and self-care intentions change.

It is important to be mindful of the temporal nature of our bodies at every stage or season, while also being exhilarated that vibrant longevity is on the rise: there are a thousand people over 100 years old in the United States alone! We witness the many forerunners of this emerging trend, such as 96-year-old vegetarian yoga teacher Tao Porchon-Lynch, who teaches every morning at 5 o'clock and shows no signs of slowing down. Or 100-year-old Australian choreographer Eileen Kramer, who told the *Sydney Morning Herald* that "everything happens at 100, everything changes."

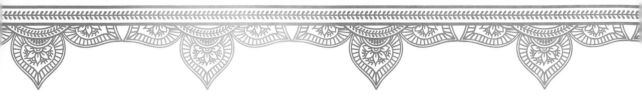

Her dancing continues as she's entered triple digits, a period she describes as "magical." These people live what biologist Bruce Lipton called the "biology of belief," which, as Dr. Christiane Northrup affirms in her 2015 book *Goddesses Never Age*, "trumps DNA." Northrup states that growing older is inevitable, though aging is optional, a result of "cultural portals," beliefs, and lifestyle choices.

Imagine if, at a young age, we knew to expect that life naturally changes and is fluid. Might we affirm and embrace our own personal life seasons more easily? Might we not be less susceptible to the next marketing campaign that tries to convince us we need to buy a new product or exotic superfood to be healthy? Might we perhaps instead be empowered to live our own authentic beauty and values, embracing tools that allow us to expand rather than those that limit us?

Many cultures accept growing older as normal, rather than seeing it as bad or harmful. In our Western culture, growing older is pathologized. We assume that we all inevitably decline, so we put in place systems to ensure that money is directed to the medical industry for curing our ills, rather than toward the wellness and beauty industry for health maintenance and pleasure healing. For me, there are many factors to sage-ing vibrantly. Aside from hair coloring, there is bodywork, movement, meditation, and daring playfulness — which is at the top of the list!

There is a season in some people's lives when coloring hair can make a difference in appearance and self-esteem; and then, for some, though not all, there seems to come a time when coloring their hair no longer provides the same result. For those who will benefit more from restoring the vibrancy of their complexion and overall vitality, regular facials are more appropriate than hair color treatments, if their budget allows for one service a month. Authentic self-observation can determine what is right for our distinctive beauty image and our personal values.

Natural wellness beauty is a journey in self-discovery. We explore to discover what it looks like for each of us, as unique individuals, to stay vibrant and sensual throughout our lives. I offer the information here as a possible lifestyle model — a viable alternative practice for coloring hair, with herbal hues.

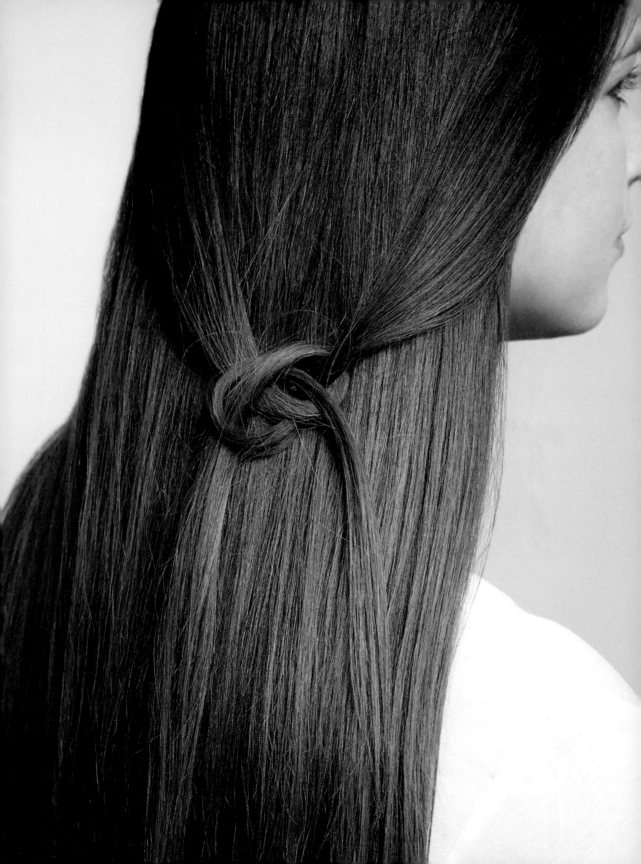

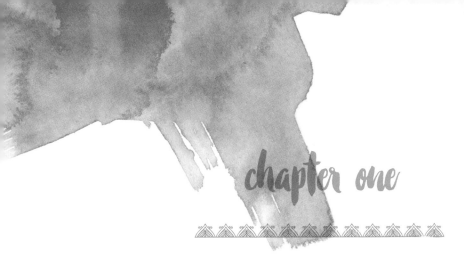

chapter one

WHY COLOR YOUR HAIR?

Attitude is the mind's paintbrush. It can color any situation.

Hair's function is to prevent heat loss from the head as well as to protect the head from heat, yet hair is such a profound part of our self-image that it causes people to spend billions of dollars each year on its care. Today, over 75 percent of American women color their hair, and this practice is rapidly growing.

What we do with our hair has had powerful symbolic and emotional effects in every culture for thousands of years. We witness the power of hair in stories, such as the one of Samson, who lost his strength when his hair was cut, and in symbols, like the live snakes that constituted Medusa's hair and were an expression of female rage. These stories and symbols speak of hair's potent ability to interface with our emotions, both individually and collectively.

Hair is an important way we express our self-image and communicate that image to others. Hair color, texture, and style preferences vary among different ethnicities and cultures, and we use hair to identify ourselves as being a part of, or separate from, these groups. I, for example, was born with coarse, curly hair typical of my ethnicity, though I straightened it through various means to fit into a culture that seemed to prefer smooth, light hair. I relate very much to the Chris Rock documentary *Good Hair*.

Entertainers change their hair to express each new project, character they play, or trending style. Our hair seems like such a simple thing, though the complexities of our human emotions make it something else!

WHY HERBAL COLORANTS?

There are many reasons why people of every age color their hair. Perhaps we do so because it is enjoyable to care for ourselves or to allow others to, or because it is refreshing to adopt a new persona. We receive tangible and intangible gifts from any colorant, so why would we want to choose herbal colorants?

> » **Herbal hair colorants connect us to ancient traditions** and generations past, and they nourish our hair, our spirit, and the earth.
> » **Herbal colorants smell "green,"** repair damaged hair, and do a better job of covering gray than chemical colors can.
> » **Pure herbal pigments are nontoxic** and can be applied frequently and remain on your hair long enough to achieve the color tones you wish without causing dryness or damage.
> » **Most people find the muds to be relaxing,** soothing, and conditioning.

Herbal colorants — especially henna — link us with the ancient past, to female nurturing traditions, to the land, and to the sun, moon, wind, and water, all of which impact these pigments. These herbal colorants also connect us with our artistic self as we blend them to create different colors.

Of the four herbs I describe in this book, the only one with a long history as a body colorant is henna. Before henna gained popularity as a hair colorant, people in hot, arid climates used it on their body as a cooling agent. Men and women would henna the bottoms of their feet to protect them from blistering when they stepped

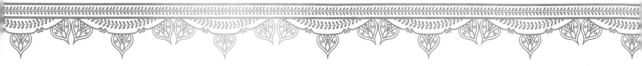

on hot surfaces. They would also henna the palms of their hands, again for cooling purposes. Out of this simple practice of staining grew the tradition of henna body art, whereby people created elaborate designs on their skin using a henna paste.

While both genders have enjoyed the benefits of henna, it is apparent that women have had a different relationship with this red-pigment-producing plant. We know that women hennaed in groups, and that the time spent together strengthened their relationships with each other and provided a short reprieve from mundane chores while they waited for the henna design to dry and set.

Henna body art is becoming more and more popular today, with the majority of henna body artists being women. Henna is often used to mark female rites of passage and special occasions, and it is currently often sought just for fun. Women's connections to sensual experiences, I believe, stem from our intimate relationships with the always-changing needs of our ever-changing bodies.

MAKING THE DECISION TO "GO NATURAL"

There are many different opinions on what "natural" means. Depending on your perspective, "natural" can mean using foods, plants, and herbs; adding supplements; or being product-free, relying instead on reflexology, yoga, and meditation to maintain your vitality.

Within this fascinating mix of viewpoints on what is "natural," I offer this perspective: nature's own ability to shape-shift and morph can be seen as a model that opens up more options for fulfilling our personal vision of what "natural" is. Part of this shape-shifting includes expanding our definition of beauty, and how we embrace and offer it to ourselves and our world.

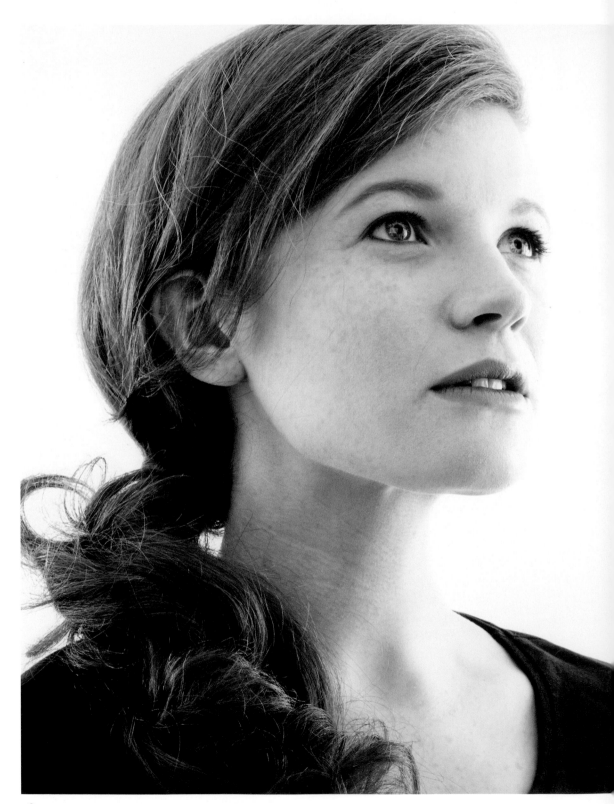

NATURAL HAIR COLORING

THE POWER OF RED HAIR

Every hair color has been known to have symbolic meaning. By looking at how people with red hair, in particular, have been treated through the ages, we see how influential the color of one's hair can be.

The term *redhead* has been used for centuries. In different eras and cultures, red hair has been either sought or feared. Across the centuries, the rarity of redheads has fueled suspicions and speculation, including accusations of witchcraft during the Dark Ages. The general opinion of redheads began to change when the vibrant natural red hair of Queen Elizabeth made this hair color seem more desirable; soon after she ascended the throne people started reddening their hair with henna.

Even today, there are mixed feelings about redheads. To celebrate their uniqueness (only 1 to 2 percent of the global population has naturally occurring red hair), redheads gather at festivals, though even presently in Britain, there are hate crimes against redheads. "Gingerism" has been compared to racism, because it targets redheaded individuals and families for harassment and violence based on their hair color.

For natural redheads who want to keep their color as they grow older, henna is an attractive alternative to chemical colorants. While it's particularly challenging to achieve long-lasting results with red chemical colorants, henna endures (especially when applied frequently) and, when combined with other herbal pigments, can reproduce the original shade of red that redheads had when they were younger.

> For natural redheads who want to keep their color as they grow older, henna is an attractive alternative to chemical colorants.

EMBRACING YOUR CRONE, EMBRACING YOUR GRAY

In our yearning for the authentic in all aspects of our lives, some of us are letting go of coloring hair entirely. Depending on your personal values and what is important to you, gray hair may be just what you want.

Men with gray hair are valued for their experience and seen as distinguished, even desirable, but women with gray hair are often devalued and seen as over the hill. The radical baby boom generation, however, is changing this image. Women who embrace their gray hair are not soft women, but rather gray-haired warriors or stunning silver foxes who are esteemed by younger sisters to the point that many in their twenties and thirties are coloring their hair gray. We know, too, people whose gray or white hair is so incredibly exquisite that we can't help but stop them on the street to affirm it! The colors of their hair, eyes, and skin combine in a way that proclaims beauty is timeless.

Part of what I do in my salon is assist those who would like to "go gray" do so with the least amount of pain. For clients with chemically colored hair, I add gray or silver highlights, alternating with lowlights, until they reach a place where they can let their hair grow out or create that ombré look. Going gray after using herbal colorants is a more natural unfolding, since the regrowth area is more subtle. It is best to simply allow the hair to grow out naturally and choose a style that will enhance the grow-out process and show off your new silver streaks.

How to Decide If Gray Is Right for You

Some people just look good no matter what color their hair is; for some, coloring their hair makes a big difference, and for others, perhaps the reality is somewhere in between. While hair color can make you appear younger, if your face sends a different message, it doesn't matter what color your hair is.

No matter your age, practice visually connecting with yourself without judgment. Doing this is such a great exercise in many ways, not the least being that it helps you make good decisions about your self-image. Try asking yourself: Is it my hair that needs coloring? Or perhaps my face needs some care? Which is my best nurturing practice for myself? Facials cost about the same as a good color treatment and, when provided by a skilled facialist, can make a world of difference in helping you be your most vibrant self. They can allow you to embrace gray hair, which may be your best look for your ethnicity, character, style, and values.

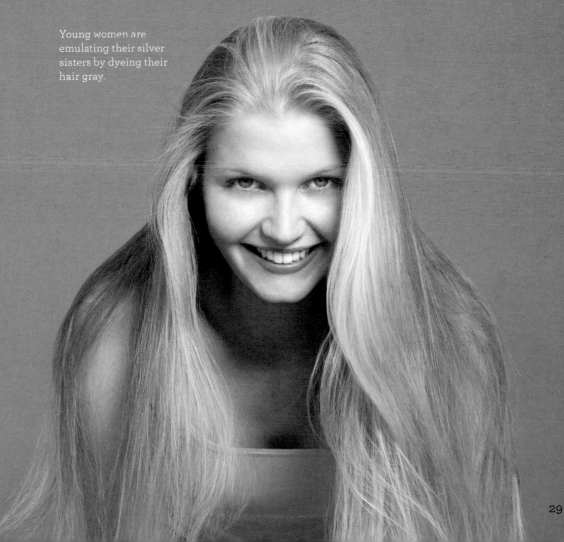

Young women are emulating their silver sisters by dyeing their hair gray.

Common Reasons We Stop Coloring

Getting off the treadmill. If we started coloring our hair fairly young, at some point we may choose to stop coloring because we've been keeping bimonthly appointments for decades and want out of that cycle. We ask ourselves: is it nurturing us?

Health issues and concerns. We need or want to stop exposing ourselves to potentially hazardous products. Doctors recommend that people stop chemical coloring when they are pregnant or ill.

Cost. The expense associated with coloring hair can be a factor. People like to switch up where they spend their money, depending on how much they have in their budget and what their values are.

Time. Herbal colorants take anywhere from 1 to 8 hours to set. If we don't want to make the time, we may choose to stop.

My Personal Gray Experience and My Return to Coloring

Like many other boom-generation women, I too did not want to miss my "crone phase." Some of my most influential role models are beautiful women who embrace themselves as gray. In 2012, I was going to embrace my crone and become a sensual sage, though I had no idea that year would hold some of my most profound transformations.

I cut my hair off instead of growing it out, and shortly after, my brother-in-law and father passed within weeks of each other. Others dear to me (10 people total) soon followed. In the midst of this, I also moved my salon, worked trade shows, juggled the demands of family and running a business, and hosted guests. Needless to say, when I finally had the space to grieve, it was, and continues to be, impactful.

Even though there was much support and excitement around growing into a new salon location, my heart needed healing. I had said from the start that I could always return to herbal colorants if I wanted, so I did. I returned to a two-step henna-indigo application monthly, though I experiment with using pure indigo alone on occasion.

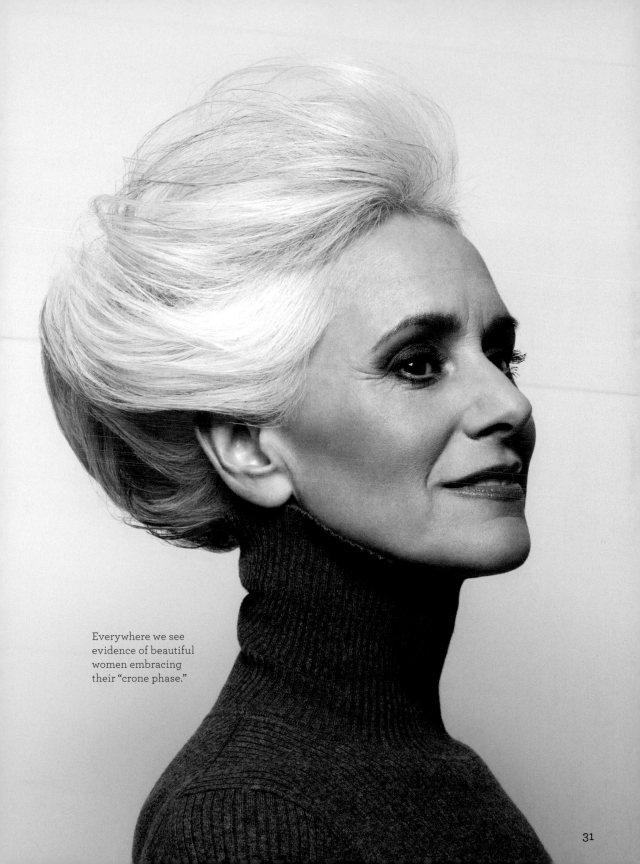

Everywhere we see
evidence of beautiful
women embracing
their "crone phase."

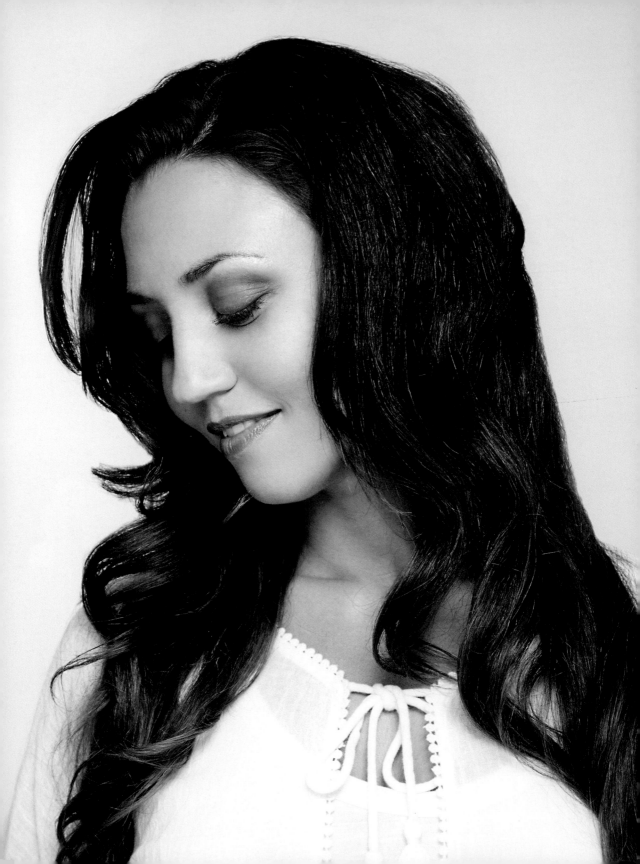

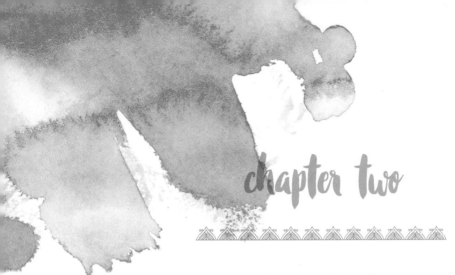

chapter two

BASIC UNDERSTANDING OF HAIR COLORING

Taking joy in living is a woman's best cosmetic.
ROSALIND RUSSELL

Hair dyeing with plants is a multicultural art practiced since ancient times. The Gauls and Saxons used various vibrant colors to distinguish rank and to enhance the battleground fear factor. Ancient Egyptians, Greeks, and Romans regularly used plant and animal matter to color their hair. There were mixes that worked with hours of sun exposure to darken or bleach hair.

Eighteen Books of the Secrets of Art & Nature, published in 1661, described the many ways of coloring hair gold, red, green, yellow, black, and even white. The colors of powdered wigs of the Baroque era ranged across an array of pastels, including pinks, pale yellows, and light blues. Bleaching hair with potassium lye or caustic soda grew increasingly popular. Women of the Victorian era wore large-brimmed hats without a top to expose their infused hair to the sun. Even gray hair was popular, and people used hair powder to enhance their gray!

The most well-known plant dyeing pigments are henna, indigo, cassia obovata, and amla. Other natural substances used in decoctions or infusions include beets, black walnut hulls, chamomile, katam, leeks, rhubarb, saffron, sage, and turmeric from the plant world, and red ocher from earth.

Synthetic dyes for hair were developed in the 1860s with the discovery of the reactivity of para-phenylenediamine (PPD) with hair. Eugène Schueller, the founder of L'Oréal, is recognized for creating the first synthetic hair dye in 1907, and in 1947, Schwarzkopf, the German cosmetics firm, introduced the first home hair coloring product. Today, hair dyeing is a multibillion-dollar industry that entails the use of both plant-based and synthetically derived dyes.

HAIR COMPOSITION AND GROWTH

Hair is unique to mammals, and human hair is intriguing because we are one of the only mammals that has areas of densely concentrated hair — on top of our heads, under our arms, and in the groin area. Human hair is also unique because of the length to which the hair on our heads will grow!

The Makeup of Hair

Hair sprouts from *follicles* in the middle layer of the skin (or dermis) of our bodies and scalp. Within each follicle is a *hair root*. The part of the hair that rises from the follicle, above the skin, is called the *hair shaft*.

> *The beauty of a woman is not in*
> *the clothes she wears,*
> *the figure that she carries or the*
> *way she combs her hair.*
> **AUDREY HEPBURN**

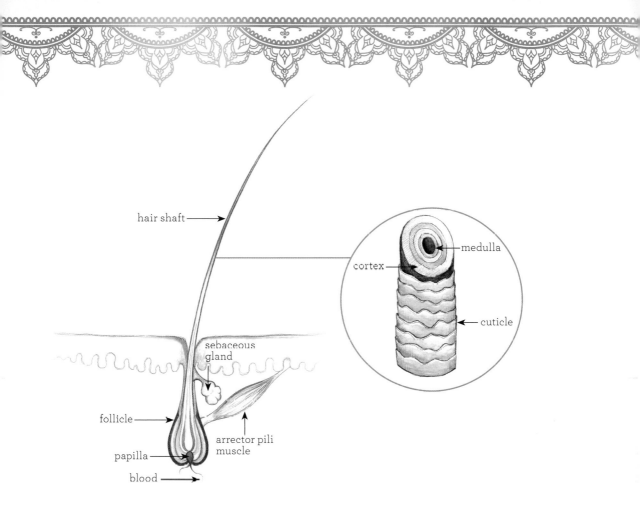

labels: hair shaft, medulla, cortex, cuticle, sebaceous gland, follicle, arrector pili muscle, papilla, blood

Hair Follicle

Within the hair follicle is the onion-shaped hair bulb in which the hair root is connected to the body's blood supply via a structure called the *papilla*. Nutrients produced in the lower part of the bulb are converted into new hair cells, and as they grow and develop, these cells steadily push the previously formed cells upward, creating "growth" of the hair shaft. The newest part of our visible hair is the part located closest to our head and is the part that most recently emerged from living cells. Stimulating blood circulation with a scalp massage helps nourish the hair and scalp.

Adjacent to the hair follicle is the *sebaceous gland* (or oil gland), which lubricates the hair to protect it and keep it healthy, and a tiny muscle called the *arrector pili*. This muscle contracts in response to a stimulus, like fear or cold, and causes the hair to stand up straight (often called "gooseflesh" or "goose bumps").

Hair Shaft

Hair is a fibrous protein made up of water, lipids, trace mineral elements, melanins, and keratin. Keratin, the main constituent in hair, is a protein created within the cortex of the hair and is very much like a rope or a cable. Built for toughness and protection, it's what makes our hair and skin waterproof. Hairs differ in cross-sectional shape. Round hairs tend to be straight; oval or flattened hairs are curly.

Each hair shaft strand has three layers (see the illustration on page 35): an outer layer of overlapping scales called the *cuticle*; a middle layer, the thickest of the three, known as the *cortex*, which also contains melanin; and usually a central core of round cells called the *medulla*, though naturally blond hair and very fine hair often lacks a medulla.

The cuticle protects the cortex from harm. When the cuticle is damaged by chemicals or physical trauma, the cortex is then exposed and open to damage. Any chemicals that are on the hair then have access directly to the bloodstream through the cortex.

HAIR FACTS

» Follicles have a cycle of active growth, transition, and rest, which includes a normal hair loss cycle called "shedding."
» Each follicle grows about 20 new hairs in a lifetime.
» Each new hair can grow to be over 40 inches long.
» Hair grows faster in warm weather.
» Hair grows more slowly at night than during the day.
» Male hair is thicker than female hair.
» Male hair grows faster than female hair.

HAIR TEXTURE AND HERBAL COLORANTS

Whether your hair is fine, coarse, wavy, curly, straight, oily, dry, normal, or a mixture of these attributes, it can receive herbal colorants beautifully. I have observed, and have heard personal testimonies, that herbal pigments tend to give volume to fine hair, tame frizzy hair, repair damaged hair, and loosen curly hair.

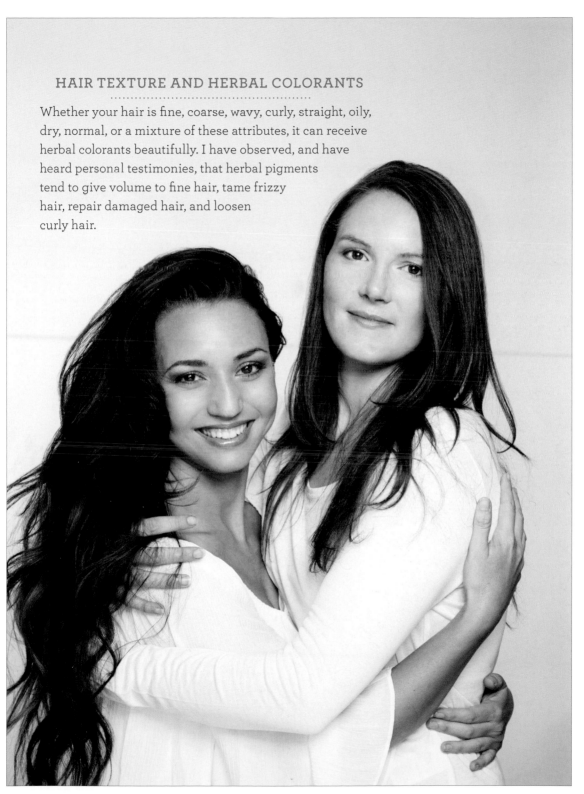

How Hair Grows

Human hair has a particular growth cycle with three different phases: anagen, catagen, and telogen. Each phase has specific characteristics that determine the length of the hair. While the phases always progress in the same order, different hairs on your head are going through different phases at any given time.

The **anagen phase** is the growth phase and generally lasts from 2 to 6 years.

The **catagen phase,** also called the transitional phase, lasts for approximately 2 weeks. During this time, the hair follicle shrinks to one-sixth of its original length and the root detaches and "rests." The hair strand is cut off from its nourishing blood supply, allowing the follicle to, in a sense, renew itself. While hair is not growing during this phase, the length of the hair shaft increases as the shrinkage of the follicle pushes it upward.

During the **telogen phase,** or resting phase, the follicle remains dormant for anywhere from 1 to 4 months. At any given time, 10 to 15 percent of the hairs on one's head are in this phase of growth. In this stage, the epidermal cells lining the follicle channel continue to grow as usual and may accumulate around the base of the hair, temporarily anchoring it in place and preserving the hair for its natural purpose without taxing the resources the body will need during the growth phase. Once the telogen phase is complete, there will be normal hair loss, known as "shedding." The anagen phase begins again, and within 2 weeks a new hair shaft will begin to emerge.

I look my best after an entire hair and makeup team has spent hours perfecting me. When do I feel my best? When I haven't looked in a mirror for days, and I'm doing things that make me happy.

ANNE HATHAWAY

REASONS FOR DAMAGED HAIR

Hair shafts can split and break in extreme situations, eventually leading to hair thinning, which is often confused with biochemical hair loss.

External factors that can cause structural damage to hair include the following:

Hair Tools: Back combing or "teasing"; combing and pulling knotted hair; excessive brushing; and overexposure to heat from too frequent use of curling irons, flat irons, or blow dryers

Chemicals: Dyeing, bleaching, perming, and frequent washing with alkaline shampoos

Nutrition: Deficiency of proteins and amino acids

Nature: Overexposure to sun and wind

What Gives Our Hair Its Color and How It Grays

Hair color is the result of proteins called *melanins*. *Eumelanin* is very dark and *pheomelanin* is lighter. The overall color of the hair comes from the various concentrations of these protein pigments. Brown and black are due to the dominance of eumelanin, and blond and red are due to the dominance of pheomelanin. Melanin levels vary over time, which is why hair color changes, and it is also why numerous colored hair follicles exist on one individual, bestowing various hair color nuances.

As hair loses melanin, it grays; white hair has no melanin at all. Bleached hair responds similarly, becoming ash or white, depending on how bleached it is. Another possible reason for color loss is that as we age, levels of an enzyme that breaks down hydrogen peroxide decline. Hydrogen peroxide, which is naturally produced by the hair follicles, builds up on the hair shaft, inhibiting melanin production. Sun exposure also contributes to loss of hair pigment.

The inability of hair to hold its own natural pigment is the basic reason why it's difficult for white and gray hair to retain chemical colorants. Anyone who has chemically colored their hair into their gray years eventually discovers that the color normally needs to be reapplied every 3 weeks, and some people need to do it more often!

HENNA AND THE SUN

Overexposure to sun contributes to loss of hair pigment, though we all need some amount of exposure. A person with moderately dark skin would do well with 45 minutes of uninterrupted sun a day, and those who are darker need more sun exposure! People with paler skin need less sun and need to be more cautious. They could use sunscreen products for hair and skin, though if not all-natural, these products can actually cause more harm than good.

Fortunately, nature has provided a natural sun block and colorant in one: henna. Coloring hair with henna protects the hair shaft from too much sun, and henna body art protects the skin.

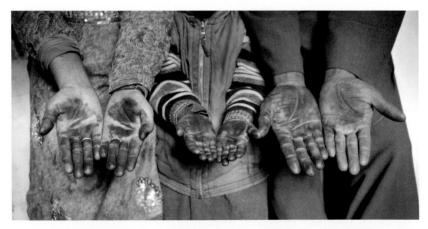

In parts of Africa and the Middle East, people apply henna on their hands and feet as protection against sunburn and chapping.

In contrast, the proteins in herbal colorants bind with the proteins in hair, making these colorants, especially henna and indigo, last longer on gray and white hair compared to chemical colorants. Herbal colorants, and henna in particular, are considered pigment "fillers" that add color where color is depleted.

Many chemical colorants use peroxide or ammonia to break down the cuticle and remove pigment before depositing the color dye molecule. Therefore, they take more quickly but also fade more quickly because the hair shaft is now damaged and cannot "hold on" to the color. Herbal tints take their time to be absorbed into the hair because they are bonding to the keratin in the hair shaft. Since no peroxide or ammonia is used or needed to break down the cuticle first, the hair is not damaged and is instead strengthened by this bond. This is a slow process, often requiring several hours of processing time depending on the condition and color of the hair as well as the color one is trying to achieve. But this extra time is worth it because once the plant color has bonded to the hair, it stays vibrant for much longer. Some of my clients do a full application of henna only once or twice a year, with root-only touch-ups in between.

CHEMICAL COLORANTS VERSUS HERBAL HAIR COLORANTS

Today, we have a vast selection of chemical hair dye colors — from normal to neon and everything between. While chemically dyeing one's hair can still cause damage to the hair, some newer lines do less damage than others. For example, the chemical hair color line I use for those clients not yet ready to jump into the herbal colorant muds is ammonia-free with a very low level (2 percent) of para-phenylenediamine (PPD). There is, and always will be, a place for chemical colorants in the beauty industry, especially as companies become better at creating these safer formulations that work with nature.

It is also important to keep traditions alive and methods for use current. There is a place for herbal color traditions, especially now, for those who need or want these options most. This includes those who are chemically sensitive, have life-threatening illnesses, are pregnant, have gray hair, are ecologically concerned, or want to live a more "organic" lifestyle that connects them with plants and their traditional uses.

Chemical Colorants

Chemical colorants remove pigment. Chemical colorants change the color of hair by breaking the cuticle of the hair shaft and changing the melanin in the cortex. The color change can be temporary, which allows the natural hair color to return gradually, or permanent, which requires either removing the new chosen color with another chemical process or applying a different colorant to change the color again. New hair grows in as its original natural color.

Chemical colorants are consistent. Chemical color formulations are consistent and readily available in most grocery stores and drugstores.

Chemical colorants are associated with toxic effects that herbal colorants are not associated with. Darker chemical colors are known to be toxic since they have more PPD (para-phenylenediamine) than lighter chemical colors. Allergies are possible and may develop suddenly, even after years of use without incident. Cosmetologists' daily exposure puts them at risk for a litany of adverse reactions, from rashes to life-threatening conditions.

Chemical colorants require frequent applications. As the percentage of gray or white hair increases, hair needs to be dyed more frequently, depending on how resistant the gray is. Many women with gray hair find themselves in a salon every 2 weeks just to maintain their hair color! Chemical colorants can also damage hair with repeated use.

TYPES OF DYES

The four most common hair color groupings are permanent, demi-permanent (deposit only), semi-permanent, and temporary.

Permanent: Permanent dyes contain an oxidizer (such as hydrogen peroxide) and ammonia. The peroxide and the ammonia open the hair shaft, affording a "blank canvas" so that the dye can actually diffuse inside the hair fiber. Dyes become trapped in the hair and cannot be readily removed through washing.

Demi-permanent: Demi-permanent hair colorants do not contain ammonia (sodium carbonate is one replacement) and contain less hydrogen peroxide than permanent dyes. Demi-permanent colorants are less effective in removing the natural pigment of hair, so they cannot make hair lighter. They are less damaging to hair than their permanent counterparts but less effective at covering gray. They wash out over time (typically 20 to 28 shampoos), and regrowth is less noticeable.

Semi-permanent: Semi-permanent colors contain no, or very low levels of, peroxide or ammonia and are therefore safer for damaged or fragile hair, though they may still contain possibly carcinogenic compounds. They partially penetrate the hair shaft, allowing the color to survive repeated washings (typically four or five shampoos). Semi-permanent colorants are affected by the hair's natural colors, creating subtle variations in shade across the whole head. As gray increases, semi-permanent colorants become less effective in blending them in with the rest of the hair color. Semi-permanent colorants cannot lighten hair.

Temporary: Temporary hair colorants do not penetrate the cortex of the hair. They coat the outside of the hair shaft with color that washes out in one or two shampoos. Temporary hair color is typically brighter and more vibrant than semi-permanent and permanent hair color, and it is most often used to color hair for special occasions, such as costume parties and theater productions.

Chemical colorants have been associated with health concerns. Some forms of cancer (including leukemia, non-Hodgkin's lymphoma, bladder cancer, and breast cancer) have been linked with the use of chemical hair colorants, though studies have not been conclusive. Here are a few ingredients that have been linked to cancer: para-phenylenediamine (PPD) and tetrahydro-6-nitroquinoxaline, coal tar, formaldehyde, DMDM hydantoin, and eugenol.

Herbal Colorants

Herbal colorants do not break the cuticle. They act more like a stain, penetrating the hair shaft and allowing the proteins of the plant pigments to bind with the hair's proteins.

Herbal colorants create a unique color. Plant pigments work with the naturally occurring color to create a color unique to you. Results vary depending on hair type, base color, and the percentage of gray in hair. Herbal colorants offer gray-haired people an opportunity to have a color with a bit of spunk, as gray hairs react to herbal pigments in unique ways. They offer this demographic an opportunity to be more playful with hair colors.

Herbal colorants make subtle changes. Herbal colorants do not drastically change your original natural base pigment; rather, they grab the lighter-pigmented and non-pigmented hairs to create a subtle change in tone and nuanced highlights. Their most basic application is brightening and enhancing normal hair color. They yield beautiful colors of strawberry, carrot, red, browns, red browns, and black! They will not turn younger hair a bright, funky color.

Herbal colorants have a longer processing time than chemical colorants. For better deposit and depth of color, herbal colorants need to stay on for at least an hour. You can also manipulate this time, leaving the muds on for shorter or longer periods, to change the depth and shade of color. By wrapping your hair in plastic and then a scarf, you can go about your business — run errands, read, garden — while your hair processes.

Herbal colorants need fewer repeated applications. The mud pigments, when used repeatedly, are more permanent than one might expect. While they will eventually wash out, on average, people go from 4 to 6 weeks between applications, depending on hair regrowth (some people can even go as long as 9 weeks between applications!).

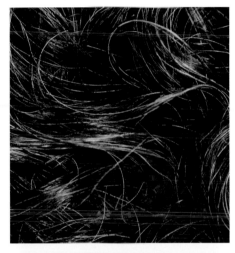

Herbal dyes create natural highlights. When herbal colorants are first applied to virgin gray hair, especially when the percentage of gray is less than that of the naturally occurring base hair color, they create a natural highlighting effect. This is a result of the variation of color tone between the light and gray hairs and base hair color.

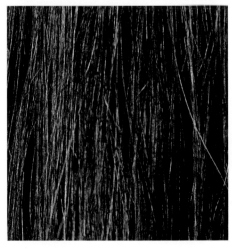

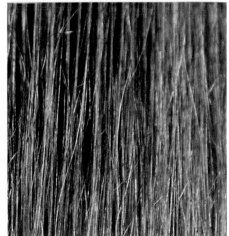

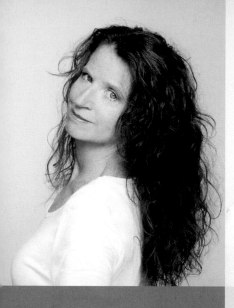

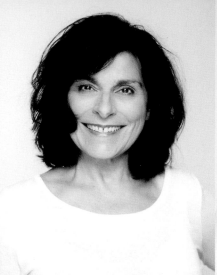

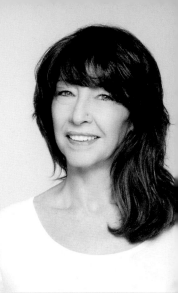

Herbal dyes can be customized. By combining different pure herbal pigments, you can develop your own "recipe" to achieve your perfect color. You can mix single herbal pigments or combine premixed commercial combinations of pure herbal colorants.

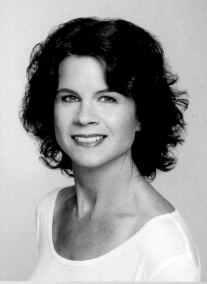

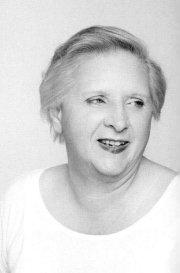

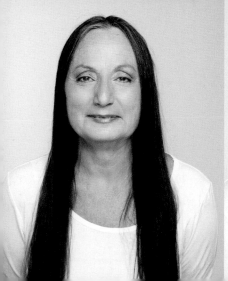

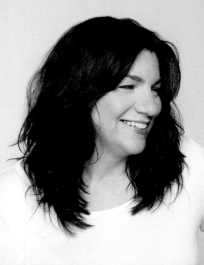

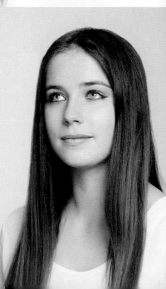

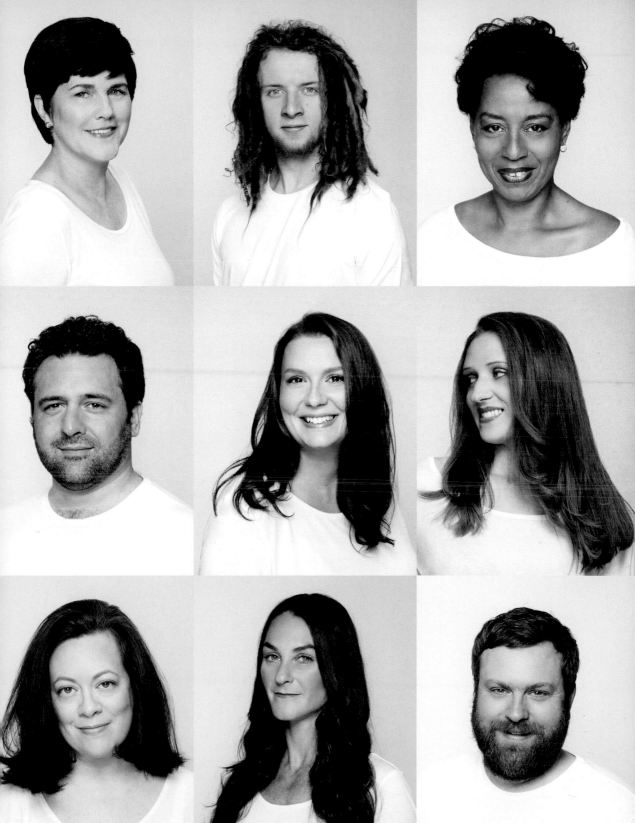

Herbal colorants show a subtle line of demarcation as new hair grows in.
Herbal mud pigments are a much better option for gray-haired individuals not yet
ready to embrace their silver years because the stain acts as a "filler," creating a
base pigment in gray hair, which no longer has pigment. As new gray hair grows in,
depending on how much, you will not see a stark line separating the gray from the
colored hair. If you have, say, 50 percent or more gray hair, the line of demarcation
at the root can be quite obvious. This is especially true if you are coloring your hair
a darker red or brown. Those with a higher concentration of gray may choose to
have their roots colored every 2 to 3 weeks.

BEFORE
(after, on
facing page)

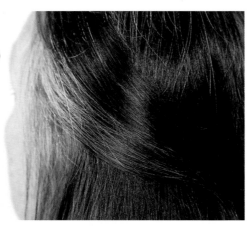

**HERBAL
COLORANT LINE:**
Note the subtle transition
from black to brown to
gray.

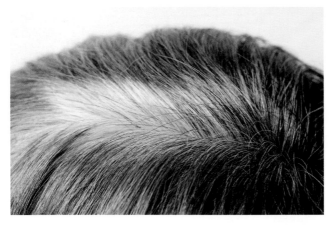

**CHEMICAL
COLORANT LINE:**
There is a stark line
separating new hair from
the chemically treated
hair.

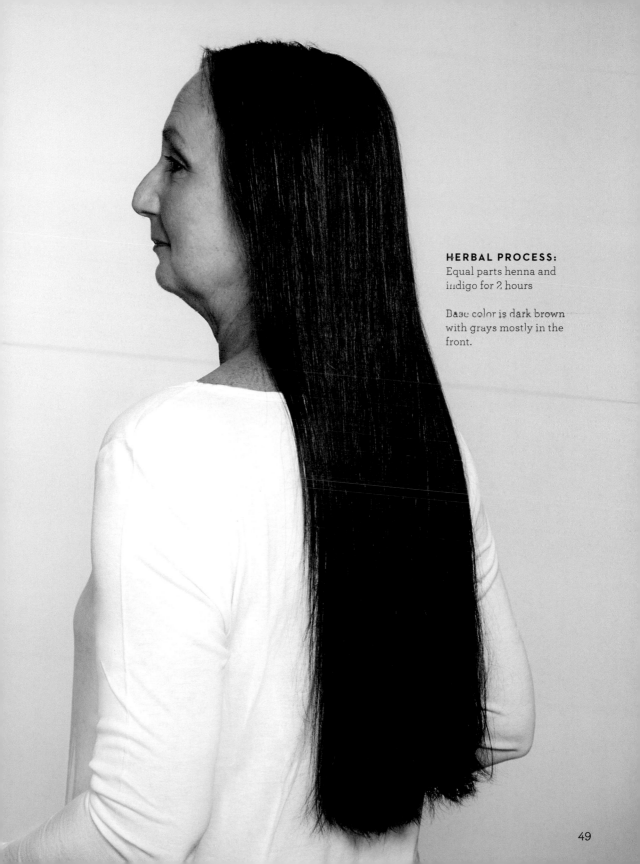

HERBAL PROCESS:
Equal parts henna and
indigo for 2 hours

Base color is dark brown
with grays mostly in the
front.

Herbal colorants do not damage hair. In fact, hair that has been repeatedly damaged with chemical colorants is restored to feeling like "real hair" after only a few applications. Hair colored with herbal pigments looks natural, rich, and authentic.

BEFORE: hair damaged from chemical color

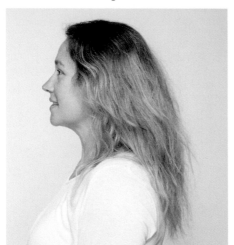 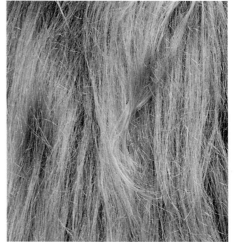

AFTER: hair texture restored and color brightened after one application (repeated applications do even more)

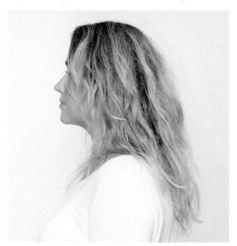 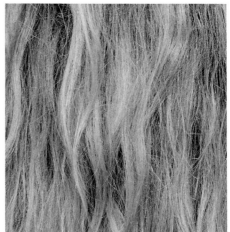

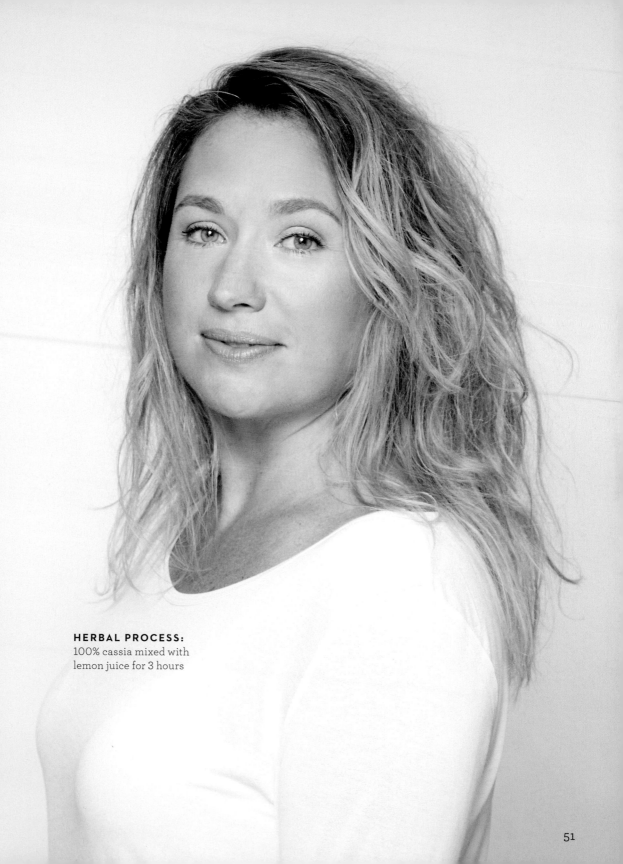

HERBAL PROCESS:
100% cassia mixed with
lemon juice for 3 hours

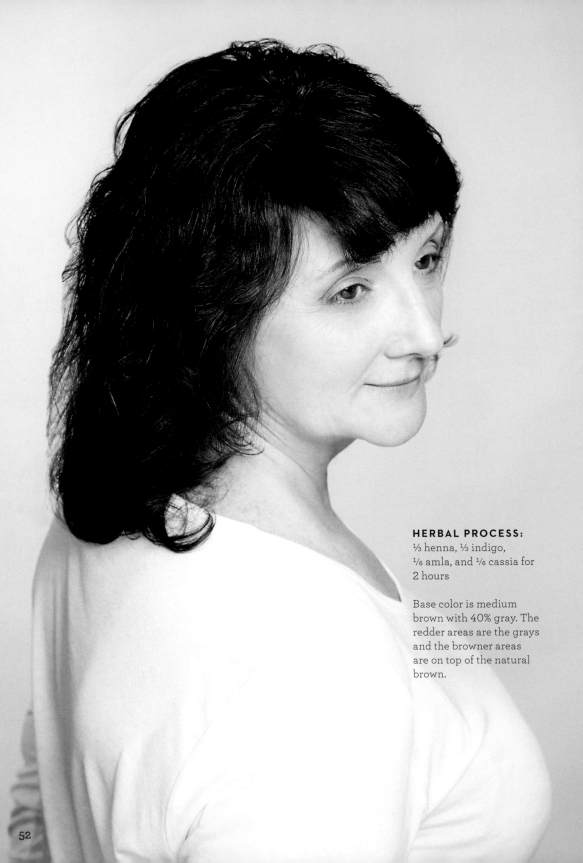

HERBAL PROCESS:
⅓ henna, ⅓ indigo,
⅙ amla, and ⅙ cassia for
2 hours

Base color is medium
brown with 40% gray. The
redder areas are the grays
and the browner areas
are on top of the natural
brown.

Herbal colorants condition hair. Hair can be fine, coarse, wavy, curly, straight, oily, dry, normal, and a mixture of these attributes. Any type will receive herbal colorants beautifully. From what I and others I have talked to have experienced, herbal colorants thicken fine hair, tame frizzy hair, repair damaged hair, and relax curly hair.

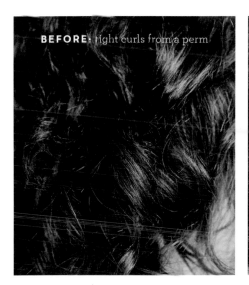
BEFORE: tight curls from a perm

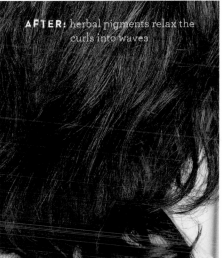
AFTER: herbal pigments relax the curls into waves

Pure herbal dyes can be applied as frequently and for as long as you wish. When powdered herbal colorants are pure, there is no limit of frequency of application; one could feasibly apply the mud daily for however long it takes to achieve the depth of color desired. There is also no time limit for keeping these colorant muds on your hair. Indigenous people who live where these plants are grown often sleep with the muds on, allowing more time for the pigment to produce deeper, longer-lasting color.

Pure herbal colorants are not toxic. Allergies are always possible with anything, though it has been my experience that they are unlikely to happen with herbal colorants. It is especially important to make sure the herbal pigment is pure. Some may actually contain adverse ingredients, such as metal salts, that can interact with other chemical treatments, or oils and waxes that may inhibit the dye, or even chemical dyes, which are common allergens. If you tend to be sensitive, do a patch test (see page 109) and remember that an allergy can develop over time.

Herbal colorants require time for "exploration." It can take some time to get the recipe right when you're first starting. Also, some herbal colorants and hair type combinations may require more processing time. Sometimes you need to apply the color more frequently, in a week or month, to achieve the desired depth and tone, and sometimes you just need to sit with the mud longer so that the pigment stains deeply. You may also need to apply a bit of creativity to certain processes, such as when you henna over chemically colored hair, at least in the beginning stage.

Herbal dyes are not always consistent. Another factor that makes it difficult to get the recipe right is that the dye content of herbal colorants is not always consistent, due to nature's unpredictable growing seasons. As with any agricultural product, the weather conditions during the growing season impact the crop's success. If the season is good, the dye content is good, and it will last for years with good packaging and storage conditions. Some years are better than others.

GOING FROM CHEMICAL COLORANTS TO HERBAL COLORANTS AND VICE VERSA

Chemical colorants to herbal colorants. Standard wisdom is to let the chemically processed hair grow out before using herbal colorants, and vice versa, but in my experience that isn't necessary. Pure herbal colorants can condition and repair chemically damaged hair. The real artistic trick is to get the line of demarcation to blend with the previously chemically colored hair. Using different colorant mediums can be tricky. Still, achieving a good blend is not impossible. It is more of a challenge to blend lighter colors than it is to blend darker ones.

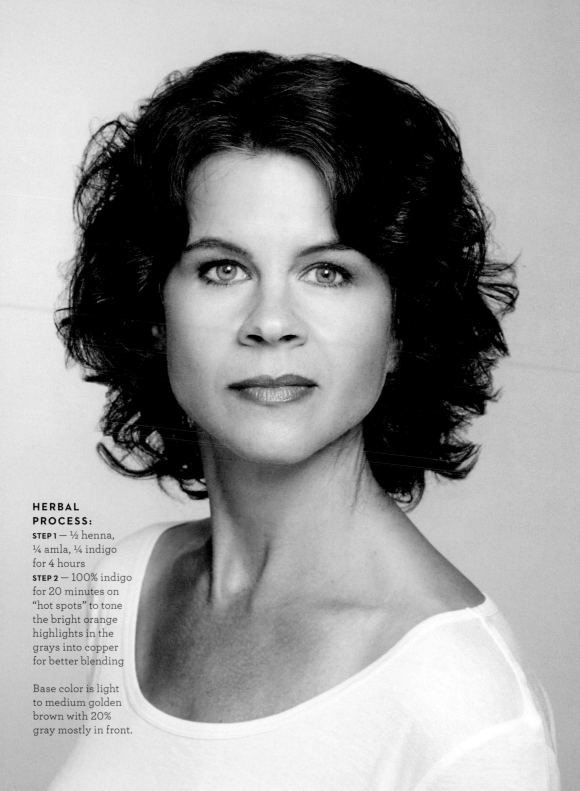

HERBAL PROCESS:

STEP 1 — ½ henna, ¼ amla, ¼ indigo for 4 hours

STEP 2 — 100% indigo for 20 minutes on "hot spots" to tone the bright orange highlights in the grays into copper for better blending

Base color is light to medium golden brown with 20% gray mostly in front.

Herbal colorants to chemical colorants. One common myth is that you can meet with disastrous results if you try to chemically color hair that has been stained with herbal colorants. In my experience, this is only true with certain products. Some store-bought henna contains metallic salts that react to the hydrogen peroxide found in chemical products that lighten hair, creating unpredictable results, such as green or blue tones. I have found that it is completely safe to use an ammonia-free chemical colorant with a low PPD content (2 percent or less) on pure herbal colorants. The hair responds normally to receiving the chemical colorant over the herbal colorant.

I have experienced no issues going between pure herbal colorants and a less toxic chemical colorant. I have even successfully used a chemical bleach cap, with a gentle bleach formulation, to help lighten hair when a henna-indigo application went too dark.

I have experienced no issues going between pure herbal colorants and a less toxic chemical colorant.

TOXIC OVERLOAD

I started coloring my hair when I was 16 years old. My best friend and I decided to try henna, so we bought henna and a bottle of wine, went home, and put mud on our heads! I remember loving how my hair felt and how shiny it was.

When I got older, I started using chemical hair colors. After many years of coloring my hair without any problems, I ended up in the emergency room with a severe allergic reaction to the hair dye. And I had been using the same product for years!

I wasn't ready to go gray, though I was still suffering from this toxic episode 8 months later, when I found Christine's salon. My first visit taught me so much about henna and other herbal colors. Christine has been doing this for quite a while, so she has lots of experience. She started with a henna-indigo blend to see if I could do a one-step process, and the result was nice — it looked more like highlights. Sometimes my grays would go green, but I didn't care because it would disappear in a couple of days, and my hair texture was improving, and I wasn't exposing myself to chemicals anymore. Then one day Christine suggested that we do a two-step process, applying henna as a gray filler and then indigo for just a short time so it would not go black, and see what we got. I agreed and have been so happy with the results! My hair color is perfect — a medium brown with some red tones — and my hair texture is so real and healthy. Everyone loves it!

Robin

ST. JOHNSVILLE, NEW YORK

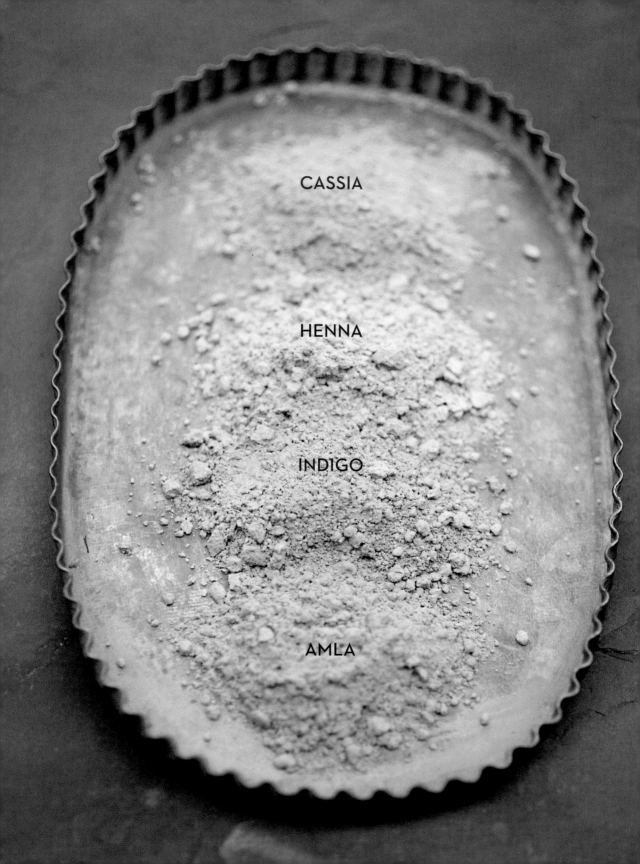

chapter three

THE FOUR PURE HERBAL COLORANTS

Finding henna is like finding a wild,
centuries-old ginseng root.

TRADITIONAL CHINESE PROVERB

My intimate relationship with these four plants — henna, indigo, cassia obovata, and amla — started over a decade ago. I began by timidly using henna on my friends and then adding indigo on my own hair. As my confidence with these two herbs grew, I turned my attention to cassia obovata for its ability to brighten and add soft blond hues and to create yellow-red tones. Lastly, I experimented with amla as a pigment adjuster to tone down the red of henna. I have since discovered that this herb has other exciting possibilities, including the ability to stimulate hair regrowth, sometimes even in shiny bald areas, and to bring color to gray or white hair without depositing a pigment.

Because three of these herbal colorants represent the three primary colors (henna is red, cassia obovata is yellow, and indigo is blue), it is easy to create custom blends for your needs. By combining these colorants in different proportions or by applying them in consecutive steps, you can achieve a wide range of colors — from blond to copper to black.

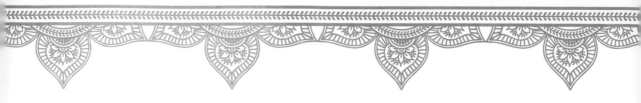

These four plants are the most common herbals used as hair colorants and can be procured easily. While this book focuses on how these herbs color hair, they each have medicinal qualities and have been used for healing for as long as they have been used for coloring — for thousands of years.

BUY ONLY PURE HERBAL COLORANTS

Some herbal colorants, particularly those generically labeled "henna," may contain adverse ingredients, such as metallic salts that could burn the hair. One henna product that I used early on in my herbal colorant journey contained green-dyed sand, perhaps to "stretch" the value of the product. You don't know what kind of filler could be added to an impure herbal colorant and what kind of allergic reaction it could cause. Always buy pure herbal colorants to lessen the possibility of allergic reactions.

Herbal colorants are native to tropical and subtropical countries with no international standard for labels. Once these products are boxed and labeled in their country of origin, they need only be exported. Because herbal colorants are considered exceptionally safe for hair, they are exempt from U.S. Food and Drug Administration (FDA) regulations, provided that they are only used as a hair colorant and meet the requirements regarding adulterants, incidental components, and labeling. This places the onus of determining whether a product is pure on us, the consumers.

When I purchase herbal colorants, I look for products that have been certified by third parties as organic, sustainable, and fair trade (see Resources, page 177, for recommened suppliers). It's hard for smaller companies to pay the price for certification, but certification can help make what can be a confusing purchase for consumers much easier.

Before you purchase a product, there are also some general signs of impurity to watch for.

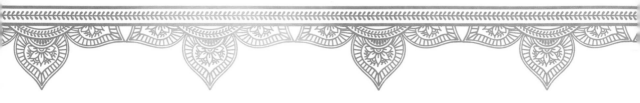

Nonpowdered form. Pure herbal colorants come in powdered form. Any product that comes in a cream, block, or paste form is likely to contain additives because once water is added, a preservative is needed to prevent microbial growth.

Use of boiling water. If the directions on the herbal colorant say to use boiling water, the herb may not be pure. Many in the henna world hold that pure herbal colorants are fragile; any boiling water can compromise the natural dye. The boiling water might be used to release metallic salts (chemical dyes) added to the herbal pigments. I have added boiling water to the pure organic henna I use and got a decent stain, though the mud was lumpy and the stain not as deep as when I use warm (not boiling) water and let the mud sit overnight for a slow dye release.

Dye release time. Pure herbal colorants require time to work. To get the best dye release, you may need to let some herbal colorants sit for at least several hours. If the directions say the herbal colorant will stain quickly, it may not be pure.

HENNA

The herb henna is the most well-known herbal hair colorant and has been used to dye hair for centuries. In the 1950s, Lucille Ball made "henna rinse" popular when her character Lucy Ricardo used it on the television show *I Love Lucy*. If you are already a redhead, color your hair red with chemical colors, or just love red hair, henna is for *you!*

Many herbal color lines sell themselves as "henna." The colors produced by these products range from red, strawberry, auburn, and mahogany to blond, brown, and black. Pure henna is always a type of red. When henna is mixed with other herbal colorants, it produces other tones, but these offerings may or may not be pure herbals.

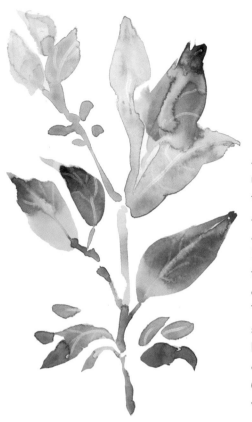

Henna the Plant

Also known as Egyptian privet, henna tree, and mignonette tree, henna (*Lawsonia inermis*) is native to the semi-arid and tropical areas of northern Africa, western and southern Asia, and northern Australasia (the region that comprises Australia, New Zealand, New Guinea, and nearby islands in the Pacific Ocean). Henna leaves produce the most dye when grown in temperatures between 95 and 113°F (35–45°C). During the rainy season, new shoots extend rapidly, producing more growth. The leaves yellow and fall during long, dry, or cool periods, and the plant dies at temperatures below 41°F (5°C). It is a midsize bushy shrub with small aromatic white or pinkish flowers and small round fruits.

SOME HENNA MYTHS DISPELLED

There is a lot of misinformation about henna in general, and this is compounded by the fact that most teachers at cosmetology schools don't know much about it. If henna is mentioned, it's usually to convey that it will burn your hair or that, if you've colored your hair with chemicals and then use henna, your hair may turn green.

In my experience, you can safely use pure henna and other pure herbal colorants on chemically treated hair, and if hair does end up with a greenish tint, you can correct it, as you would if a chemical color went green or ashy. Pure henna will not burn your hair. Pure henna always conditions, improving and actually repairing damaged hair. If hair is burned with henna, it's because the henna has been adulterated with metallic salts or some other additives.

History of Henna's Use as Dye

Henna is world-renowned for its beautiful red dye. Henna has been used throughout history to dye everything from skin, hair, and fingernails to fabrics — including silk, wool, and leather. It has been used as a cosmetic hair dye for 6,000 years. People of ancient Egypt are known to have dyed their hair with henna, and people in other parts of North Africa, the Horn of Africa, the Arabian Peninsula, the Near East, and South Asia have been using henna for centuries.

Mehndi is the term used to refer to henna body art, which has been used in beauty rituals and customs from time immemorial, due to the association of its red coloring with good luck and general auspiciousness. It has also been used in rite-of-passage ceremonies for pregnancy, birth, weaning, puberty, circumcision, marriage, and even death. Henna is the oldest recorded cosmetic and has been widely used

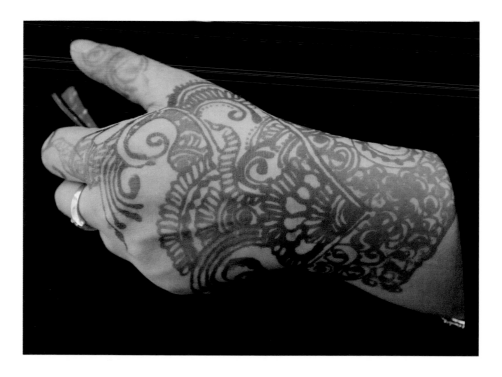

by people from all over the world and of different religious beliefs and ethnicities. Many sacred texts from various faiths throughout the world reference henna. Any hot, dry region where henna is grown usually has henna traditions.

Because henna's use was so widespread, its specific date or country of origin is difficult to pinpoint. Inscriptions place henna in Syria as early as 2100 BCE. There is evidence that Greeks used henna for applications such as mehndi around 1700 BCE and that henna was in use during the Egyptian dynastic periods around 1500 BCE. Beautiful cave paintings made with henna have been found in Ajanta, India, and date back to 400 BCE.

NEUTRAL AND BLACK "HENNA"

"Neutral henna" and "black henna" do not contain any henna. They come from other plants, or from other questionable substances entirely.

"Neutral henna" comes from the plant cassia obovata, which is also known by its Latin name *Senna italica*. It is called "neutral" and categorized as a nonpigment because the deposit is subtle and takes repeated use to yield hues. It is used mostly for conditioning hair and for therapeutic applications or for creating custom herbal hair color. The leaves of cassia obovata are also ground, making a light green powder that "smells green."

"Black henna" powder may have indigo (*Indigofera tinctoria*) as its source, but it may also contain dyes and chemicals. *Caution:* "Black henna" may contain para-phenylenediamine (PPD). This chemical stains skin black, but it's dangerous: it sometimes causes severe allergic reactions and permanent scarring.

Henna Color

Pure henna stains hair red, orange, or a rich red brown, depending on your natural base hair color and the quality of the henna. Henna can be mixed with other natural hair dyes, including cassia obovata, for lighter shades of red or even blond. When mixed with indigo, it produces brown and black shades. Some products sold as "henna" include these other natural dyes.

Conventional beauty wisdom says that henna is a temporary color, but it's actually semi-permanent. In my personal experience using henna for nearly a decade on myself and others, I've learned that while henna can fade over time and wash out, it usually takes a long time to do so. Furthermore, if you continue to color every month or two, the color will grow richer.

Henna that is used for body art is higher in dye content than henna typically sold for use on hair. I only use body art–quality henna. The leaves come in powdered form and boast a scent of grass or hay.

CAUTION: *If you have a G6PD deficiency, avoid using henna. It could produce serious health problems. Talk to your doctor for more information.*

Traditional Medicinal Uses

Henna's bark and seeds have been used for therapeutic purposes in the ancient medicines of Unani and Ayurveda for centuries. One of henna's main properties is that of a cooling agent, so it is applied to burns and scrapes and is often used to treat heat exhaustion or the fever of a sick person. It is used topically on rashes and fungal infections, including athlete's foot and ringworm. Henna is a complete sun block. If you tan with your mehndi body art, as the red color fades, a white pattern remains where your mehndi was!

Henna has also historically been used to treat severe diarrhea caused by a parasite (amoebic dysentery), stomach and intestinal ulcers, cancer, enlarged spleen, headache, jaundice, and skin conditions. It is often applied directly to the affected area for dandruff, eczema, scabies, fungal infections, and wounds. Many henna users attest that scalp issues they had had for years disappeared after their first try with henna.

Henna essential oil, or absolute, has a tea-like bouquet and a delicate note of sweet licorice. This henna oil can be mixed with the dye, and both prevent skin infection. Henna leaf absolute is now mostly used for perfumes and biblical blends.

HOW TO TEST IF YOUR HENNA IS PURE

Once you've purchased henna, there are a few tests you can run. Here's how to tell if your henna is pure:

» **Glass Test:** Rub a tiny bit of henna between two pieces of glass; if there is a scratching sound and/or the glass scratches, sand has been added, a technique used by some companies to stretch their henna powder to make more profit.

» **Bright Green:** If your henna powder is bright green rather than yellow green, and a green dye instead of a red brown dye pools around the mud once it has been mixed and set, a green dye has been added. Do not use! It is not pure henna.

» **Fizz Test:** Coat hairs taken from your brush with 1 teaspoon of prepared henna mud and let stain for at least 1 hour. Mix 1 ounce of 20-volume hydrogen peroxide with 20 drops of ammonia in a small bowl, and add the dyed hair to the mixture. If nothing happens, you have pure henna! If the hair strands turn green, melt, boil, immediately change color, or smell nasty (not like grass), then *do not* use! Most likely, the henna has been tainted with metallic salts.

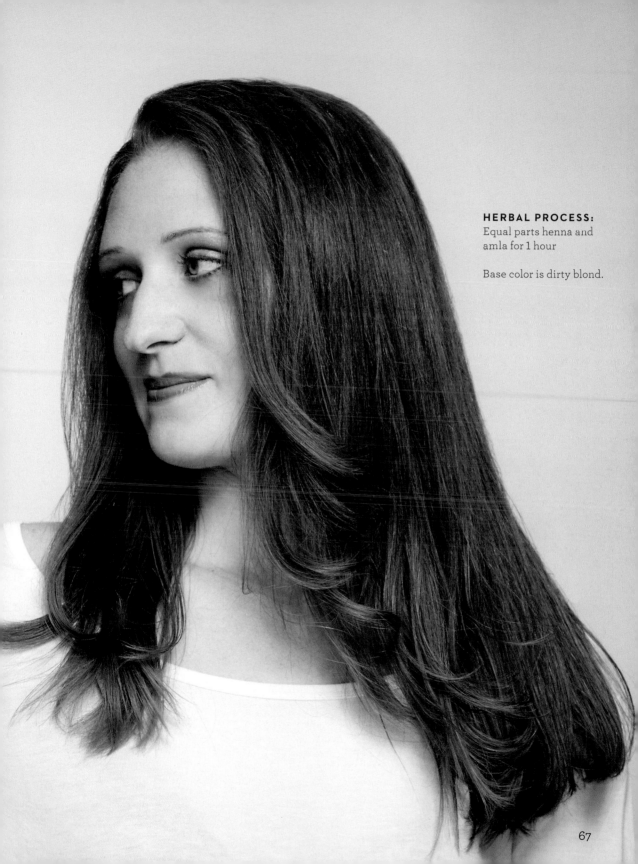

HERBAL PROCESS:
Equal parts henna and
amla for 1 hour

Base color is dirty blond.

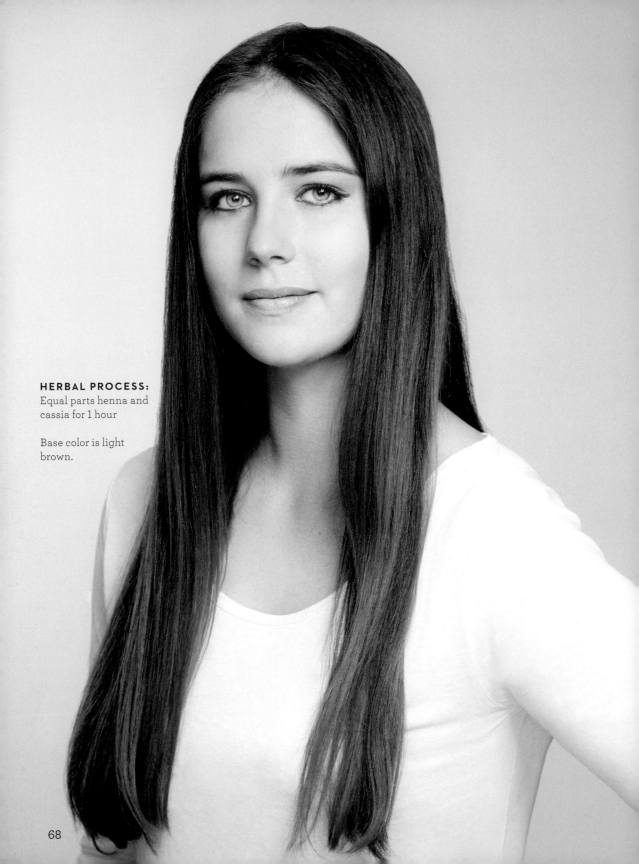

HERBAL PROCESS:
Equal parts henna and
cassia for 1 hour

Base color is light
brown.

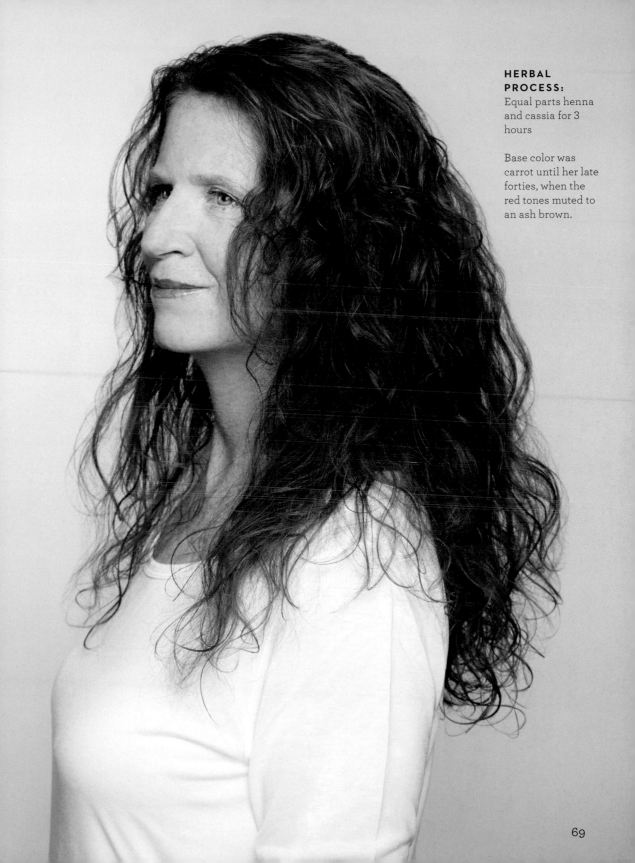

HERBAL PROCESS:
Equal parts henna and cassia for 3 hours

Base color was carrot until her late forties, when the red tones muted to an ash brown.

69

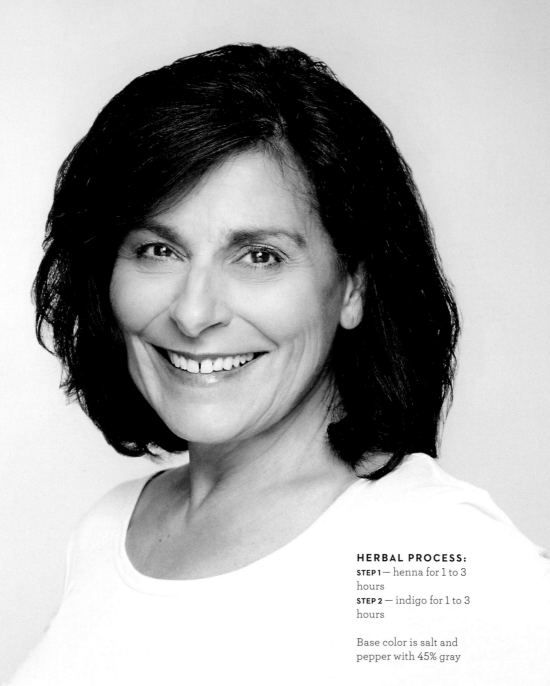

HERBAL PROCESS:
STEP 1 — henna for 1 to 3 hours
STEP 2 — indigo for 1 to 3 hours

Base color is salt and pepper with 45% gray

NOT ALL WHO WANDER ARE LOST

My name is Elaine, and I am a mud head. I was born with black, curly, shiny hair. As I began to gray, I colored with chemicals and needed to reapply every 4 to 5 weeks. I never liked the look of a white scalp next to newly colored hair; it didn't look natural. Plus, I started getting bumps, thinning hair, and sore spots on my scalp with each coloring.

I wandered into Faces of Astarte one day because the words "natural hair coloring" and "no chemicals" caught my eye. Christine's space is unlike any salon I'd ever seen; it is elegant and inviting, and its subtle aromas are very welcoming.

An application of henna and indigo did the trick. My scalp was soothed after the first treatment, and unsolicited compliments abounded. The color is a natural-looking, shiny, rich dark brown with auburn hues. And the hair thinning has stopped!

My regrowth is not the stark skunk look of white next to colored hair, affording me more weeks between coloring.

It has been 18 months since I became a mud head, and I color my hair every 5 to 6 weeks in the comfort of my home. I schedule an appointment with Christine to dye my hair every third or fourth time as a treat for me, and to touch base with her.

At home, I first apply the henna and let it stain. After I rinse out the henna, I apply the indigo and leave that in for 1 to 1½ hours to achieve the color I like on my regrowth. The whole process takes a total of 3 hours. This time is my downtime to do whatever: listen to music, clean, read, catch up with long-distance friends, watch a movie, or just relax.

Christine's continuous availability as a resource when I have questions is comforting. The henna/indigo experience has made a positive difference for me, thanks to Christine.

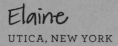

UTICA, NEW YORK

INDIGO

Indigofera tinctoria, common name true indigo, was one of the original sources of blue dye; woad was another. Indigo has naturalized to tropical and temperate Asia and parts of Africa. It has been cultivated for many centuries worldwide, and its native habitat has not been determined. While most dye today is synthetic, natural dye from indigo is still available and promoted as a natural coloring.

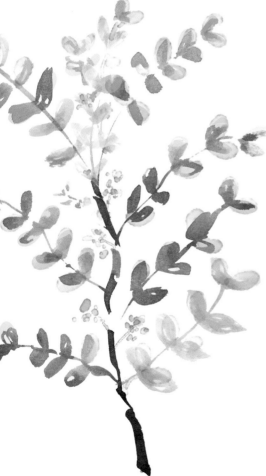

Indigo the Plant

True indigo is a shrub that is 3 to 6 feet high. It may be an annual, biennial, or perennial, depending on the climate in which it is grown. It belongs to the quite large plant genus *Indigofera,* which boasts over 750 species. True indigo has light green feathery leaves with bundles of pink or violet flowers and is a legume. Like other legume crops such as alfalfa and beans, it is rotated into fields to nourish the soil.

History of Indigo's Use as a Dye

Indigo is among the oldest dyes to be used for printing and dyeing textiles, and India is the oldest known center for indigo dyeing. For the past 4,000 years, indigo has also been used to color hair.

Northern Europeans were slow to adopt indigo as a dye source, because they had long relied on a blue-pigment-producing plant called woad (*Isatis tinctoria*) for that purpose. Since Roman times, woad had been cultivated extensively in northwestern Europe. The people of the British Isles used woad for many centuries: Ancient Celtic people used it to dye their bodies blue to frighten foes. In England, Robin Hood and his men achieved the Saxon green color of their clothing by dyeing their clothes in woad and a yellow plant dye called wild mignonette (*Reseda luteola*). Over time, woad became a major industry and trade item.

It is easy to see how unrest ensued when merchants tried to introduce indigo to Europe, which woad merchants called "devil food." An international political group of woad producers called the Woadites formed to ban indigo. England, France, and Germany passed laws prohibiting indigo importation. In the sixteenth century, Dutch, Portuguese, and English traders brought indigo to Europe from India. Gradually, indigo replaced woad as the preferred dye in western Europe. The British dropped all obstacles to indigo trade when they occupied India and began the East India Company.

HOW TO TEST
IF YOUR INDIGO IS PURE

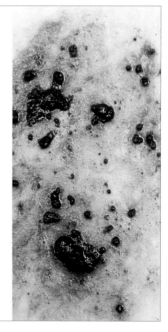

When pure indigo is mixed with water and allowed to sit for 10 to 20 minutes, a blue glaze appears on the surface, though the inner mud remains closer to green. To test the purity of an indigo powder, put a pinch of it on a very wet paper towel and wait about 15 minutes for a colored liquid to separate away from the towel. If the liquid is greenish blue, the powder is pure indigo. If it's yellowish green, it's real indigo but it may have a low dye content. If the liquid is black or brown, the powder contains chemical dyes and you should not use it.

In North America, indigo was introduced to colonial South Carolina. There, it became the colony's second most important cash crop after rice, with much if not all labor performed by African slaves.

Indigo Color

The leaves of the indigo plant contain its famous deep blue dye. Production of the dye entails harvesting, drying, and grinding the leaves into powder.

For coloring hair, combine indigo with henna to achieve deep reds, brown reds, browns, and black. You can mix dry indigo into already marinated henna (or mix indigo with water and then add to henna) and add the combination at once to hair. Or you can perform a two-step process in one of two ways: you can first stain hair with henna and then stain it with indigo, or you can do two consecutive stains of the henna-indigo mixture, the first time for fill and the next for color.

I have used indigo alone on pure white hair, and it first turned an amazing bright green and then became an amazing deep purple in a few days! If you like to celebrate St. Patrick's Day and you have all-white hair, you might want to try pure indigo.

Traditional Medicinal Uses

Ayurveda and other traditional medicine systems use indigo to address a number of ailments, such as lung issues including asthma and bronchitis, as well as cancer, depression, hemorrhaging, and problems with the spleen and kidneys. Other traditional medicine systems in India have treated cardiovascular and urinary tract problems with indigo. Some of these healing traditions also recommend placing a paste made with indigo leaves on sores and ulcers and applying a decoction of the leaves to burns and the stings and bites of venomous creatures to relieve pain and quicken healing. Traditional Chinese medicine relies on indigo to reduce fever and inflammation, to cleanse the blood and liver, and to relieve pain.

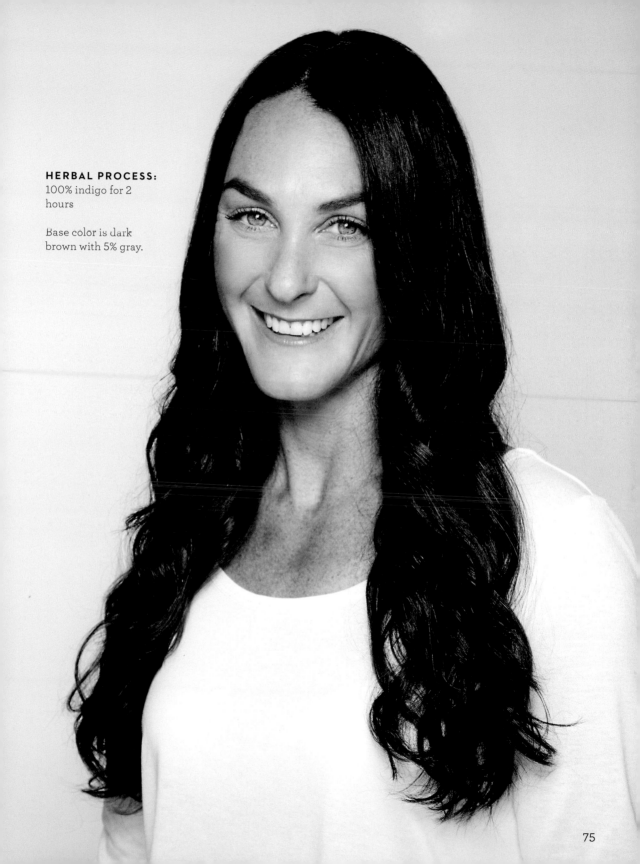

HERBAL PROCESS:
100% indigo for 2
hours

Base color is dark
brown with 5% gray.

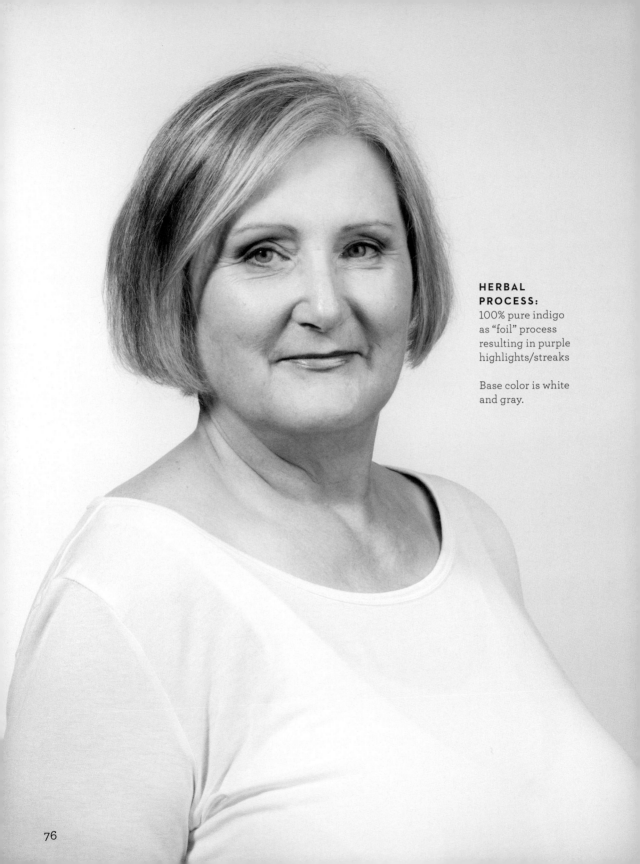

HERBAL PROCESS: 100% pure indigo as "foil" process resulting in purple highlights/streaks

Base color is white and gray.

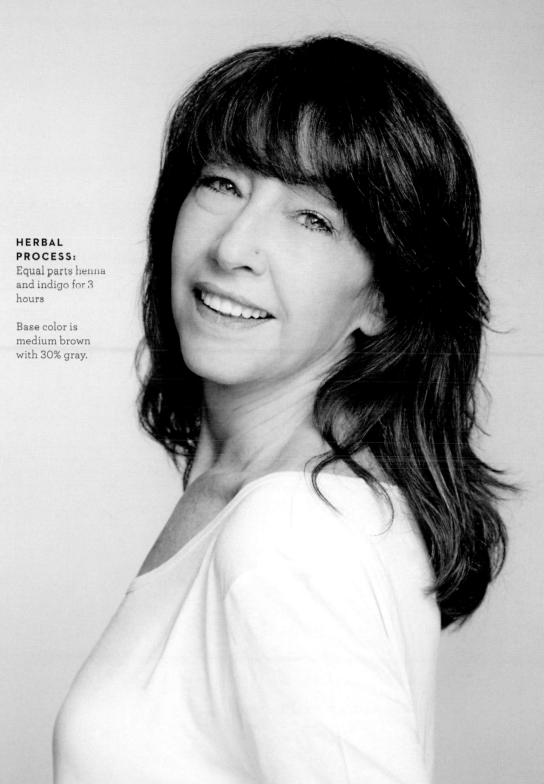

HERBAL PROCESS:
Equal parts henna
and indigo for 3
hours

Base color is
medium brown
with 30% gray.

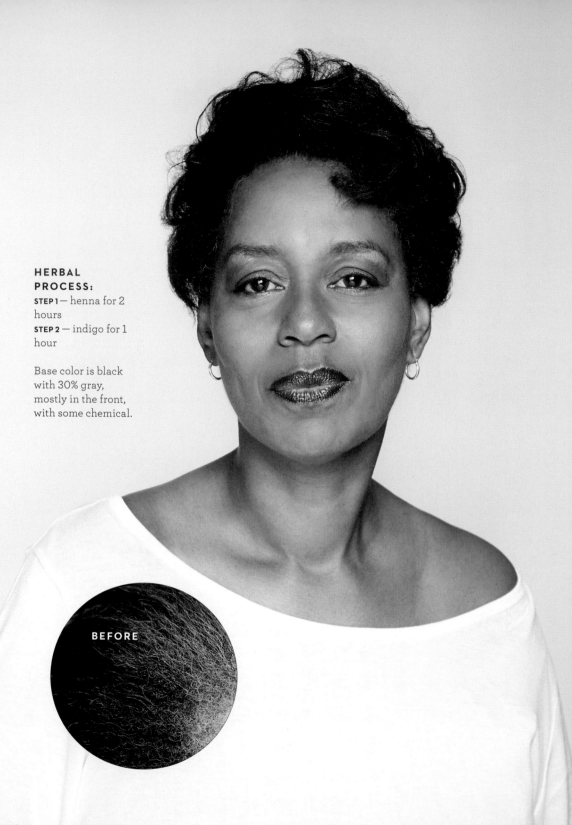

HERBAL PROCESS:

STEP 1 — henna for 2 hours

STEP 2 — indigo for 1 hour

Base color is black with 30% gray, mostly in the front, with some chemical.

BEFORE

AMLA

While we use the leaves of the other three herbs, it's amla's fruits that are dried and used on hair. Not traditionally known as a colorant, amla is most often used in combination with other herbs to adjust tone. Amla is also a very important herb in Ayurvedic medicine and has many healing properties.

Amla the Plant

The amla tree (*Emblica officinalis*) grows in central and southern India, Burma, and Ceylon. Furrowed light green or yellow fruits sit on short stems closely set along its branches. Its simple feathery leaves shade the fruit; its flowers are also greenish yellow. The fruits, most commonly known as Indian gooseberries, ripen in autumn and are hand-collected by harvesters who climb to the upper branches where they grow. Indian gooseberries are sour and bitter. In India, people commonly steep them in salt water and turmeric to make them more palatable.

While they share the same name, the Indian gooseberry and the commonly known European gooseberry are not related. The Indian gooseberry is a tree and its fruit contains a big stone, while the European gooseberry is a bush whose fruit has many small seeds. Though acclaimed as the "new super-fruit" by those in the Western world of dietary supplements and alternative medicines, the amazing amla/Indian gooseberry is ancient and was written about in the *Rig Veda*, a collection of religious hymns that was recorded in approximately 3000 BCE.

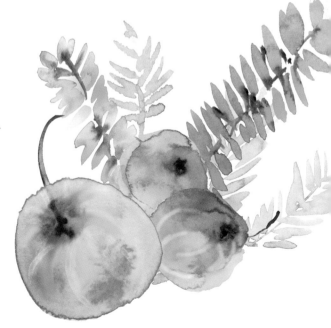

Amla Color and Benefits

Amla is most often used as a color adjuster to tone down the red of henna. While most resources indicate that amla does not color hair on its own, in my experience it enhances natural hair color. I have seen amla create a cool brown tone when used alone repeatedly on a natural brown base color, and a beautiful champagne color on all-white hair.

A most exciting benefit from amla is that it brings color back to gray and white hair, and it stimulates hair growth. It also strengthens hair roots and boosts color and luster, due to its carotene and iron content. Its general antioxidant capacity protects hair follicles from free radical damage and the hormones that can cause hair loss.

There are two ways you can combine amla with henna to adjust color: You can add powdered amla directly to the premixed henna, mixing until smooth, and add water if needed to adjust the consistency. Or you could mix amla with water until you have a smooth paste, and then add it to your prepared henna paste. The ratio of amla to henna depends on the amount of red tones you desire. For more red, use more henna; for less red, use more amla.

To use amla alone for hair therapy, make a mudpack from amla powder and water (some people add yogurt or oil) and massage into the scalp; then wrap the scalp with plastic wrap and a warm towel or thermal cap. Allow the mudpack to stay on the scalp for anywhere from 15 minutes to several hours. I usually have clients sit with it for an hour, then wash and condition as normal. You will see the color enhance immediately, though the color will continue to develop over time with regular use. When using amla for hair regrowth, I have witnessed new downy hairs growing in shiny bald areas after a couple of hair treatments.

Amla brings color back to gray and white
hair, and it stimulates hair growth.

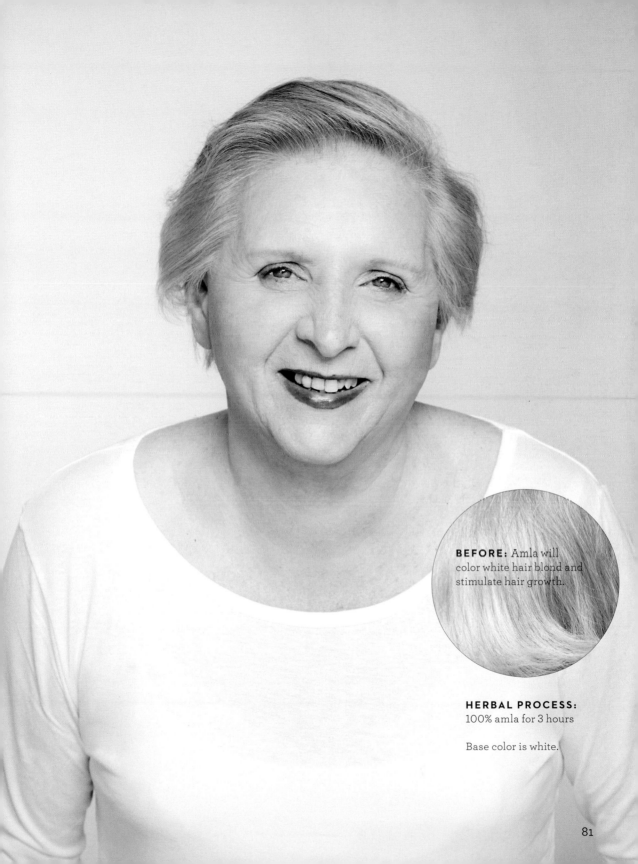

BEFORE: Amla will color white hair blond and stimulate hair growth.

HERBAL PROCESS:
100% amla for 3 hours

Base color is white.

Traditional Medicinal Uses

Amla is a sacred tree for Hindus, as Vishnu (one of the three supreme deities of Hinduism) is believed to dwell here. The tree is worshipped on a specific lunar date in February known as Amalaka Ekadashi, which is also another name for the tree. Tree worship is a common practice of Hinduism, which maintains that the Universal Spirit or Omnipresent God resides in everything.

Another reason Hindus venerate this tree is that its medicinal qualities seem endless. Every part of the tree is useful, and the fruit in particular is a common ingredient in Ayurvedic therapeutic formulations. Amla contains copious amounts of natural tannins and vitamin C.

Pure powdered amla purchased for use on hair is safe to ingest. The powder can be mixed with juice to make a healthy tonic. According to Ayurveda, amla balances all three doshas (mind-body types that express particular patterns of energy). Amla is unique because it contains five of the six tastes fundamental to Ayurvedic practice. Ayurveda recommends it as a rejuvenative to promote longevity and to strengthen the heart, benefit the eyes, stimulate hair growth, enhance digestion, alleviate constipation, reduce fever and coughs, cleanse blood, alleviate asthma, and enhance intellect.

Amla is also a traditional beauty treatment. Regular use of amla strengthens hair follicles, stimulates hair growth, stops hair loss, boosts hair volume and curl, prevents premature graying, remedies dandruff, prevents split ends, and nourishes hair! Its history as a traditional beauty enhancer includes use as a facial scrub and toner, and today it is a popular ingredient in shampoos and hair oils.

CASSIA OBOVATA

Senna italica is the Latin name of the tree whose leaves are used to produce cassia obovata, a colorant used to dye hair. (I will refer to it as simply "cassia" from now on). The plant has no relation to the cassia cinnamon tree (*Cinnamomum cassia*), the source of the spice used in cooking.

Cassia the Plant

Senna italica (also called Senegal senna, Italian senna, or Port Royal senna, depending on where it is grown) is native to West Africa, North Africa, Sudan, the Horn of Africa, and the region from Yemen to northwest India, though it has naturalized in some parts of South Africa. The tree can grow to be up to 2 feet tall and has feathery leaves. It is adapted to warm temperatures and may grow throughout the year. The yellow or orange flowers of *Senna italica* are bisexual and bloom mostly during the rainy season, but flowers can blossom year round in moist surroundings. Fruits are oblong or ellipsoidal. The dried leaves and pods of Senegal senna are traded for medicinal uses. Dried and powdered leaves from Egypt or India are traded internationally as hair conditioner.

Cassia Color

Chrysophanic acid is the name of one of the antimicrobial substances the various species of *Senna* share. In its pure form, chrysophanic acid is yellow, and in high concentrations it can stain skin and hair a yellow tone; therefore, it is often referred to as "blond henna" (which by now you understand is a misnomer because henna produces only red tones). It is also referred to as "colorless" or "neutral henna" because cassia does not change the pigment of hair that has a dark base color. Unlike chemical blond colorants, cassia does not "lift" hair tones, but for those with lighter shades of hair such as dirty blond, blond, strawberry blond, or even bleached hair, cassia will add brightness and color to the natural blond hues, which will deepen with repeated use. When used on gray hair, it will "tone down" the silver and gray shades.

I also use cassia in combination with the other herbal colorants to adjust shading. Cassia combined with various amounts of henna creates different shades of strawberry blond and red (such as copper and carrot). Combined with indigo, it brightens and/or lessens the ash tones on gray hair. It can also produce shades of browns when combined with henna, amla, and indigo. Further, it is a splendid hair conditioner, adding shine and thickness — and contributing to a happy, healthy scalp!

Both cassia and henna are green powders. While they look similar, a trained eye can tell the difference: cassia is a yellow green while henna is olive green.

Traditional Medicinal Uses

There are four hundred species in the genus *Senna*. Many of the *Senna* species are used in Ayurvedic, Unani, and folk medicines as antifungals, antibacterials, and laxatives. Ninth-and-tenth century Arabic pharmacopoeia noted their effectiveness against what we now recognize as microbes and fungi.

Senna alexandrina has largely replaced *Senna italica* for medicinal purposes. However, *Senna italica* remains in wide use within domestic markets as a mild laxative ingredient.

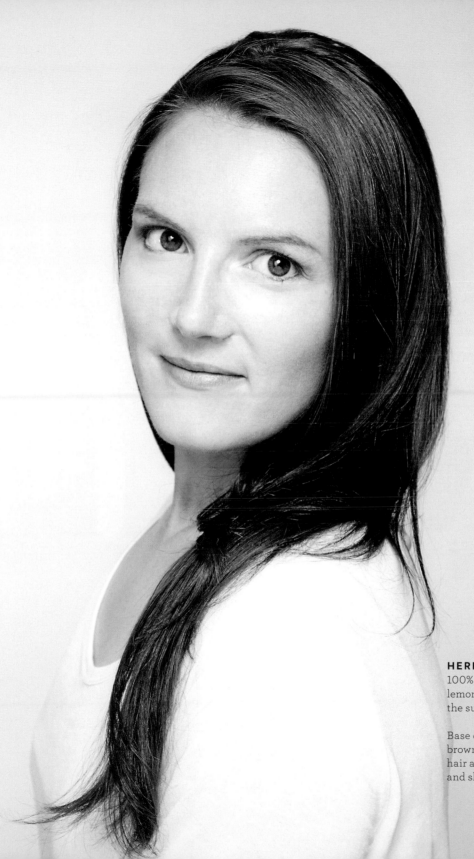

HERBAL PROCESS:
100% cassia mixed with
lemon juice for 2 hours in
the sun

Base color is medium
brown. Cassia conditions
hair and adds brightness
and shine.

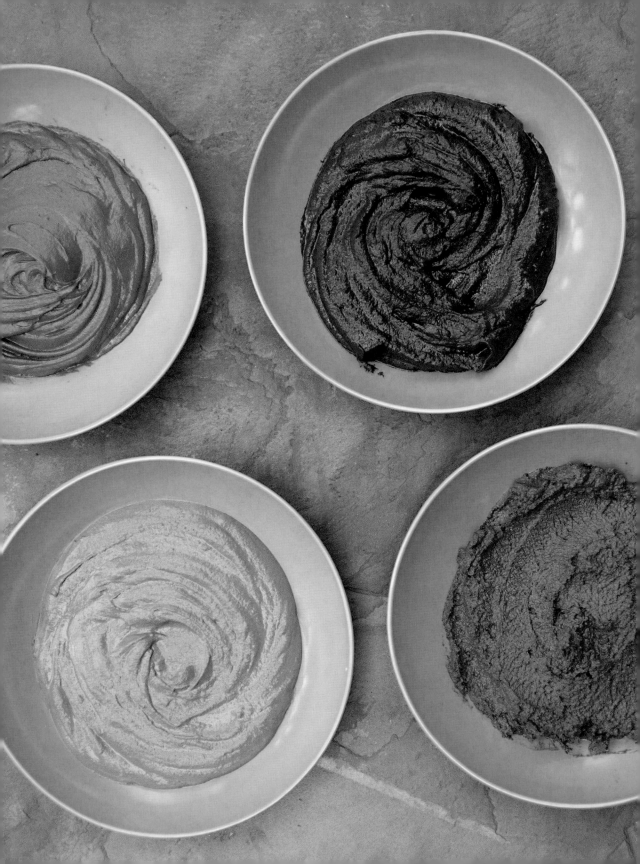

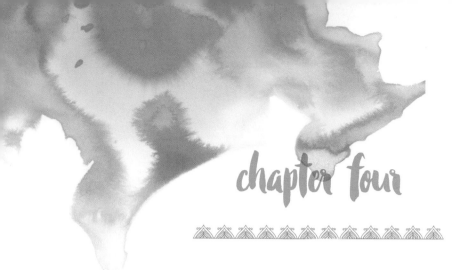

chapter four

HOW TO USE HERBAL HAIR COLORANTS

My love affair with nature is so deep
that I am not satisfied with being a mere
onlooker, or nature tourist.

EUELL GIBBONS

The recipes and application information that follow are gained from my personal experience using henna, indigo, cassia, and amla daily in my salon/spa Faces of Astarte. The basic coloring process is simple: select your color recipe; mix the pure powdered herb(s) with a liquid to form a mud; apply the mud to your hair; wrap your mudded hair in plastic and a covering; let the stain work for at least 1 hour; rinse out the mud; and then shampoo, condition, and style as usual.

Within this basic framework, there is much room for adaptation and creativity. While there is always a level of experimentation when using herbal hair colorants, in time, by applying the basic principles I outline here, you can create your perfect color recipe and learn how to adapt it as needed. And, perhaps more important than that, you will have fun tapping into your creative artistic side as you explore these earthy muds and nourish yourself. Time to jump into the mud!

CREATING YOUR COLOR RECIPE

Hair colored with herbal pigments looks natural, rich, and authentic. Herbal colorants perform beautifully on all types of hair, and they will yield beautiful colors of strawberry, carrot, red, brown, red brown, and black.

Depending on the color result you want, you may be able to use just one pure herbal colorant. If not, you will want to mix different herbal colorants together to create your perfect shade. Which herbs you select, and in what proportions, will be your "recipe." See the chart on pages 92–95 for guidelines.

Hair colors can be broken down into categories, allowing for a better understanding of what can often be confusing definitions. The first step is to determine your base color, whether it's natural or from a previous hair coloring treatment. The second is to identify your color tone (warm, cool, or neutral).

Identifying Your Base Color

Whether or not you use chemical colorants, the color of your hair at this moment is your base color. To use the recipes on pages 92–95, identify your primary base color (dark brown, dirty blond, carrot, and so on) and go from there. If you want to go a little deeper, or you just want to explore the fun of creating your own recipe, try taking a closer look at your hair.

It may seem like a simple thing to identify your base color — "I'm a dark blond" or "I'm a redhead," you may be thinking — but remember back to our discussion of melanin in chapter 2. Melanin levels vary across your head, producing different colors and shades of coloring. To get a sense of the variations in your color, just take a section of your hair and look at each of the individual strands, or if your hair is short, go outside into natural light with a hand mirror and study the hair reflected there. For example, while your hair may look "carrot-colored" overall, when you examine individual strands you will see that some hairs are deep red, some are white, and some are carrot. Herbal pigments will stain each of these colors differently, so by being

aware of the different colors on your head and their rough proportions (medium brown with 10 percent gray with blond highlights, for example), you can get a better sense of which herbal pigments you need to create a certain look.

Determining Your Color Tone

There are three underlying color tones: warm, cool, and neutral. A simple way to determine yours is to consider which color clothes you look best in.

Warm Tones

People with warm coloring look best in gold- and copper-colored clothes, and their skin has a yellow undertone. If you look better in gold than silver jewelry and look better in peach than pink, then you are probably warm. Here are some typical warm-colored skin and eye color combinations:

- » Golden blond hair, fair skin, and blue eyes
- » Golden brown hair, fair skin, and hazel eyes
- » Black hair, golden olive skin, and brown eyes
- » Red hair, fair skin, and brown or hazel eyes

When considering hair color, think bronze, copper, or golden, which add warmth to your hair color. The herbal colorants that produce these tones are henna and cassia.

The ugly duckling is a misunderstood universal myth. It's not about turning into a blonde Barbie doll or becoming what you dream of being; it's about self-revelation, becoming who you are.

BAZ LUHRMANN

Cool Tones

People with cool coloring look best in blue and violet colors, and their skin has a pink undertone. If you look better in silver than gold jewelry and look better in navy than tan, you are probably cool. Typical cool-colored skin and eye combinations include the following:

» Dark hair, fair skin, blue eyes
» Blond hair, fair and rosy skin, and blue eyes
» Black hair, very dark to black skin, and deep brown eyes

When considering hair color, think ash, champagne, or platinum, which add coolness to your hair color and are often used to tone down brassiness. For herbal colorants, use amla and indigo.

Neutral Tones

Those who are neutral-toned have both cool and warm undertones (some have more of one than the other). Those with neutral tones can wear all or most colors of clothes and jewelry. Because they have both cool and warm tones in their skin, hair, and eyes, there is a wide variety of hair colors that could work for them.

My Recipe Guidelines

I have confirmed age-old recipes on my herbal hair coloring journey and then experimented with incorporating the tried-and-true basic color theory used in chemical hair coloring procedures. The chart that follows is the culmination of my years of experience and research. Don't feel that you need to stop with my recipes, though. Creating herbal colorant mixes is a personal journey. Talk to people who color their hair with these herbs and you will learn that they each have their own unique preparations and preferences.

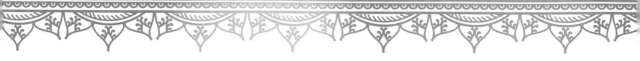

After you try a recipe, it's a good idea to record your results. Try writing down the recipe you used and describing the resulting color, and your feelings about it, in as much detail as you can. This will help you decide which recipe to use or how you need to tweak your current recipe the next time you're ready to color.

Allow yourself some time to find which recipe works best for you. You could find the right combination of herbal colorants right away, or it could take you a few tries, though it should not take longer than that. With experience, the time gap between where you are and where you want to be gets shorter.

SOME LIMITS OF HERBAL COLORANTS

There are three basic tones in herbal colorants: red, yellow, and blue. These are all you need to begin an herbal colorant journey, and other plant pigments can be added as your experience grows. Still, plant pigments produce a narrower range of tones than chemical colorants.

Unlike chemical colorants, herbal colorants cannot lift or lighten dark hair. The best results come from repeated use within a family of color, such as strawberry, copper, red, red brown, dark brown, and black. Cassia, the blond-hued herbal colorant, will brighten all hair colors when used in various amounts but only stain gray, white, or naturally light blond hair over time.

Also, herbal colorants won't turn pigmented hair bright funky colors, such as teal, green, or purple. What's exciting, though, is that they can have this effect on white or gray hair. This offers those with non-pigmented hair an opportunity to be a bit more playful with hair colors — an option the baby boom generation just may want to explore!

MY HERBAL COLORANT RECIPES

The color ratios I suggest here are for virgin hair — hair that does not have a line demarcating chemically colored hair from natural, new growth. If you do have chemically colored hair with a line of demarcation, you can still use these ratios, but you will then need to use some ingenuity and instinct to create a second recipe to blend that line of demarcation (see page 117 for more information).

HAIR COLOR GOAL	BASE COLOR	HERBAL COLORANT RECIPES
Blond hues 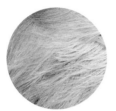	Blond, dirty blond, gray, or white	100% pure cassia (*Remember: cassia is not bold, so longer staining time and more frequent applications are advisable*) *or* 100% pure amla (*as pictured; quicker result*)
Brighter tones 	Any color, though the change is more obvious on light and medium brown, blond, and white	HERBAL COLORANT RECIPE 100% pure cassia
Strawberry hues 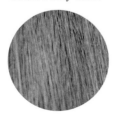	Blond, dirty blond, gray, or white	HERBAL COLORANT RECIPE ¾ pure cassia ¼ pure henna

HAIR COLOR GOAL
Carrot hues

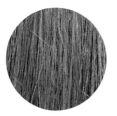

BASE COLOR
Blond, dirty blond, gray, or white

HERBAL COLORANT RECIPE
½ pure cassia
½ pure henna

HAIR COLOR GOAL
Copper hues

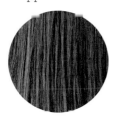

BASE COLOR
Blond, dirty blond, gray, or white

HERBAL COLORANT RECIPE
½ pure cassia
¼ pure henna
¼ pure amla

HAIR COLOR GOAL
Red hues

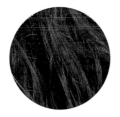

BASE COLOR
Blond, dirty blond, gray, or white

HERBAL COLORANT RECIPES
½ pure henna, ¼ pure amla, ¼ pure cassia

or

½ pure henna, ½ pure amla

or

100% pure henna

HAIR COLOR GOAL
Cool red hues

BASE COLOR
Medium or dark brown

HERBAL COLORANT RECIPES
½ pure henna
½ pure amla

or

½ pure henna
¼ pure amla
¼ pure indigo

HAIR COLOR GOAL Red/brown hues 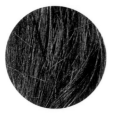	BASE COLOR Medium or dark brown	HERBAL COLORANT RECIPES ½ pure henna, ¼ pure cassia, ¼ pure indigo *or* **Step 1:** 100% pure henna for 1 hour **Step 2:** 100% pure indigo for 10 minutes or more if needed
HAIR COLOR GOAL Copper/brown hues 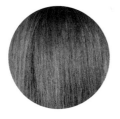	BASE COLOR Medium or dark brown	HERBAL COLORANT RECIPE ⅓ pure henna ⅓ pure amla ⅓ pure cassia
HAIR COLOR GOAL Light brown 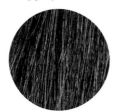	BASE COLOR White, blond, or red	HERBAL COLORANT RECIPE ½ pure henna ½ pure indigo *If you need more brown tones, do a two-step application of the henna-indigo mixture. Or next time mix ⅓ pure henna with ⅔ pure indigo.*
HAIR COLOR GOAL Medium brown 	BASE COLOR Brown or brown with moderate gray	HERBAL COLORANT RECIPE ⅓ pure henna ⅓ pure indigo ⅓ pure cassia

HAIR COLOR GOAL
Basic dark brown

BASE COLOR
Medium brown,
dark brown, or black

HERBAL COLORANT RECIPES
⅔ pure indigo, ⅓ pure henna

or

Step 1: 100% pure henna
for 1 hour
Step 2: 100% pure indigo
for 20 minutes

HAIR COLOR GOAL
Warm dark brown

BASE COLOR
Medium brown,
dark brown, or black

HERBAL COLORANT RECIPE
⅓ pure henna
⅓ pure amla
⅓ pure indigo

HAIR COLOR GOAL
Cool dark brown

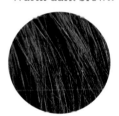

BASE COLOR
Medium brown,
dark brown, or black

HERBAL COLORANT RECIPE
⅓ pure henna
⅓ pure amla
⅓ pure indigo

HAIR COLOR GOAL
Black

BASE COLOR
Any color

HERBAL COLORANT RECIPE
Step 1: 100% pure henna
for at least 1 hour
Step 2: 100% pure indigo
for at least 1 hour
*(Note: The longer the indigo is
on, the darker the black.)*

Creating Your Own Recipe

One great benefit of herbal colorants is that you can create your own custom color. To create your own recipe, begin by looking at the chart on pages 92–95 to get a sense of what works together, and then experiment for yourself.

When making your recipe, keep in mind basic color theory: the primary colors (red, blue, and yellow) are the only hues that can't be created by mixing other colors together. Henna is red, indigo is blue, cassia is yellow, and amla varies depending on base color, since amla is not a pigment to be added but rather a tone adjuster. By mixing these herbal colorants together, you can create various shades of blond, red, and brown, as well as black. Use the color wheel on page 98 as your guide.

The primary color wheel is the color mixing chart we were taught in elementary school. It was designed by painters for painters in the eighteenth century to show how mixing the three primary colors of red, blue, and yellow created secondary colors (orange, purple, and green).

The shoe that fits one person pinches another; there is no recipe for living that suits all cases.

CARL JUNG

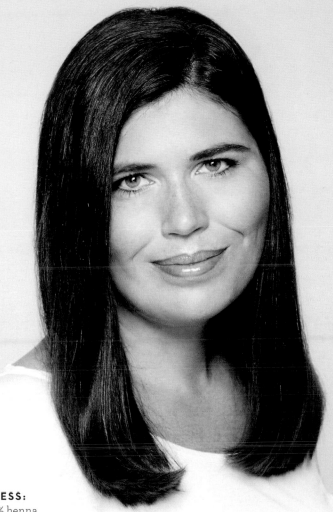

HERBAL PROCESS:
95% cassia and 5% henna

Base color is medium golden brown with red undertones and 3% gray.

Henna added color to grays that resisted cassia's deposit.

We know that by mixing red and green, we create brown, but by mixing blue and orange, as well as many other color mixtures, we also produce brown! Achieving a brown color is fairly simple; obtaining an exact shade of brown takes more intention.

All colors cover an extensive range of tones and shades. Light, medium, and dark browns, for example, contain warm and cool tones — bluish, greenish, yellowish, and reddish — that create particular browns.

COLOR MIXING WHEEL

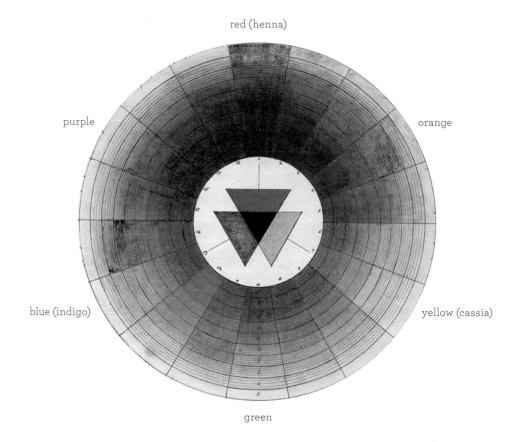

red (henna)

purple

orange

blue (indigo)

yellow (cassia)

green

MOTHER TO DAUGHTER

I've been coloring my hair naturally with a henna/indigo mix for the last few years. My natural color can be best described as mud puddle brown. I never appreciated my natural color, so as a young adult in my early twenties, I sought to change it. I've always adored auburn red hair, so auburn was generally my color of choice, which I accomplished using various salon and over-the-counter chemical products. After coloring my hair for so many years, by the time I started going gray I was burned out on the whole yucky chemical coloring process. So, I chose to let my hair go gray. But because I was mostly gray in the temples and a little on top, the natural look really didn't work well for me. Thank goodness I was able to try henna with a knowledgeable beauty goddess, Christine Shahin.

Not only does henna/indigo color my hair a rich auburn chestnut, but the shine and thickness are superior to chemical coloring. I also adore the "instant highlights" I get. Rather than a full monotone color, the henna/indigo mix penetrates each hair shaft, maintaining the natural-looking varied highlights we all desire. I'm more than pleased with my experiences with henna, and I am looking forward to using it until I am ready to embrace a full head of silver locks.

I introduced my 7 year-old daughter to the all-natural henna experience when she told me that she wanted red hair like Anna from the Disney movie *Frozen*. I never would have used a chemical color on her, but I also didn't want to patronize her without considering her desire to have red hair. I thought henna would be a great option for her because it's all-natural and good for the hair. Her color looked beautiful, with such rich, natural tones. She received many compliments on her hair, not just because of the gorgeous color but because of the shine and thickness. My young picky daughter wasn't in love with the smell, so she hasn't wanted to color again; however, it was a great introduction to herbal colorants. When she's older and ready to play around with her hair color again, I bet she'll choose henna.

Kimberely
NEWPORT, NEW YORK

MIXING AND STORING

All of the pure herbal colorants that I use come in powdered form and need to be mixed with a liquid (either water or an acidic liquid, depending on the herb) before they can be applied to the hair. Amla can be mixed in advance and left to set overnight, or it can be used immediately after mixing without waiting; indigo needs to be used immediately after mixing; henna and cassia release their dyes slowly and need to be mixed at least 2 hours before application, or preferably mixed in advance and set overnight.

Influences That Can Affect Stain

Each herb naturally contains a different amount of the key staining ingredient. Many things can affect the level of this constituent, including climate and soil as well as how the colorants are processed and stored and how long they remain in storage.

Also important is the temperature of the mix when you set your herbal colorants. Temperature affects the rate of dye release, and therefore saturation levels. Liquids added to the pigments can be at room temperature or warm. Some people say that you should never use boiling liquid to mix your colorant, believing this could compromise the pigment; I myself have used boiling water on pure henna and gotten a good stain, but the mud was lumpy rather than smooth and the stain not as deep. In the foothills of the Adirondack Mountains where I live, the weather can get very cold, yet still I "keep it simple, sweetheart" and don't fuss with incubating (warming the mixture while it sets). I mix henna and cassia, which release their dye slowly, in a plastic container, covered only with its lid, and let the color develop overnight before applying it to hair. I repeatedly get a very good stain.

Materials for Mixing

I so love the vase that sits on my mixing table holding wooden spoons and plastic spatulas stained with the pigments of the herbal colorants I mix. The process of coloring has left my tools feeling organically hand-stained, connected, and imprinted.

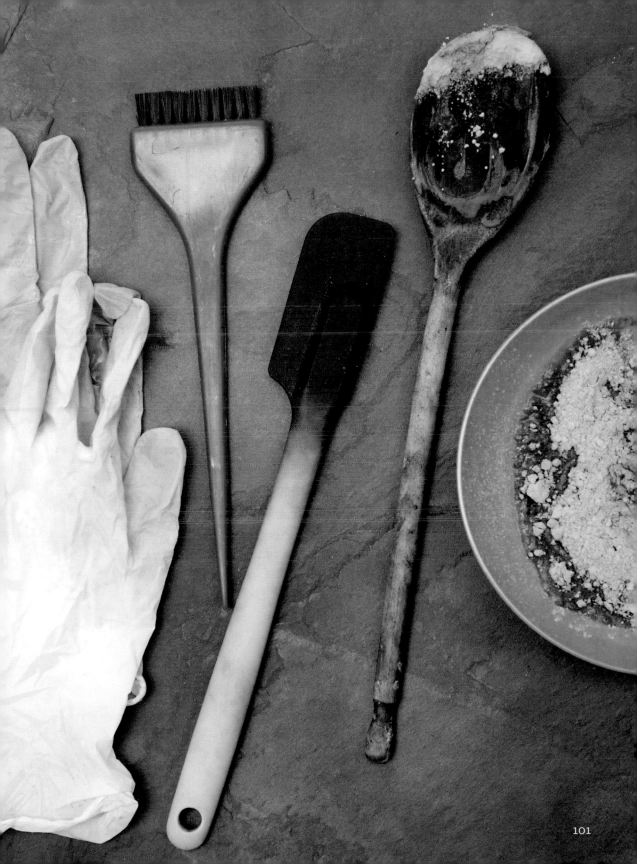

CASSIA

HENNA

INDIGO

AMLA

When I mix amla or indigo for immediate use, I mix only what I need and usually mix the mud in a plastic or ceramic bowl. When I mix the slow-release pigments henna and cassia, I use plastic tubs with tops so these colorants can sit for the required hours undisturbed and protected. I have also mixed slow-release pigments in stainless steel and ceramic bowls with no issues, though glass and plastic containers with sealing lids are more appealing for their convenience. Avoid using aluminum bowls and containers, since aluminum is a reactive metal and we don't know what it could do to affect the process.

MATERIALS TO HAVE ON HAND

FOR MIXING

» Spoons (wooden, plastic, or stainless steel)
» Mixing bowls (ceramic, plastic, glass, or stainless steel)
» Glass or plastic containers with tops (for henna and cassia)
» Room-temperature or warm water (for amla and indigo)
» Acidic liquid such as lemon juice or apple cider vinegar (for henna and cassia)
» Coffee, black tea, or herbal tea such as lemon or raspberry (optional)

FOR APPLYING

» Old T-shirt or sweatshirt (for wearing when applying the mud)
» Towel set aside for use with herbal colorants
» Thermal cap (optional)
» Gloves (if working with henna or indigo)
» Paintbrush or plastic application bottle (optional)
» Plastic wrap or plastic bag (to wrap around mudded hair)
» Hair wrap, skullcap, or scarf (optional; to cover plastic to keep head warm, or for a more appealing appearance while in public)

Though I generally do have specific containers for my pigments, these herbal colorants are also medicinal herbs, so I do not have concerns about using the same bowls to mix colorants as I use for my food. It's a beautiful thing to not worry about toxic contact, isn't it?

How to Mix Henna and Cassia

For best gray coverage, mix henna and cassia with an acidic liquid, such as apple cider vinegar or lemon juice, to help the pigment adhere to hair (I have also used plain water in a pinch with no adverse effects). If I'm looking to add yellow, I favor adding lemon juice, and if I'm adding red, apple cider vinegar.

You can also experiment with mixing henna and cassia with various other liquids such as coffee or teas, alone or in combination with apple cider vinegar or lemon juice (see box on opposite page). The main criterion to consider when choosing tea is how the color of the tea will combine with the herbal colorant. Lemon juice or chamomile tea mixed with cassia will add a boost of brightness to cassia's blond result. Similarly, adding lemon juice or chamomile tea to henna will brighten henna with a hint of gold. Conversely, using raspberry or pomegranate tea and apple cider vinegar will give cassia and henna a red assist.

Add liquid to the pure herbal powder until the mixture is the consistency of pudding (see photo at right). For example, if you're using 3½ ounces (100 g) of powder, start with ½ cup of liquid, stir, and add more as necessary to make a thick pudding consistency. The amount of powder you need varies by hair type and length (see box on page 106). Then cover the mixture and let it sit, undisturbed, for several hours (at least 2 hours; overnight is best). Henna does seem to be a bit lumpier than cassia, but after sitting for several hours, the lumps in the henna will disappear with stirring.

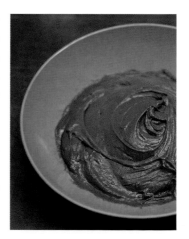

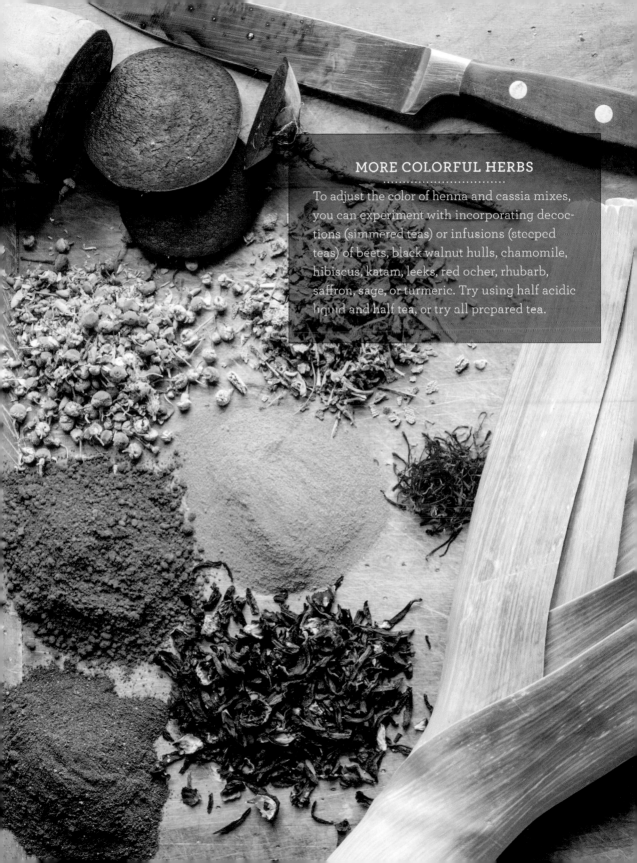

MORE COLORFUL HERBS

To adjust the color of henna and cassia mixes, you can experiment with incorporating decoctions (simmered teas) or infusions (steeped teas) of beets, black walnut hulls, chamomile, hibiscus, katam, leeks, red ocher, rhubarb, saffron, sage, or turmeric. Try using half acidic liquid and half tea, or try all prepared tea.

Some people prefer to add a few drops of an essential oil with a scent they like (such as lavender or geranium) or a few kitchen spices (such as cinnamon, cardamom, or cloves), but these are not necessary for improving the stain on hair. Still others love the distinctive earthy aroma of the herbal colorants.

HOW MUCH POWDER?

The amount of herbal colorant you need to color your hair will depend on your hair's length and thickness and if you will be coloring the regrowth area or the length of the hair shaft. If mudding your entire head, you will generally need about 1¾ ounces (50 g) for chin-length hair and 3½ to 7 ounces (100–200 g) for long hair.

How to Mix Amla and Indigo

Indigo is most potent when used immediately. Indigo and amla are mixed only with water. Sometimes I use slightly warm tap water (not hot and never boiling), as I believe the warmth gives the mud a smoother texture than when using cold water straight from the tap. Again, the amount of water you need will vary by the amount of powder you are using (see box above), but as a guide, if you're using 3½ ounces (100 g) of powder, start with ½ cup water, stir, and continue to add more water as needed until you have a thick pudding texture.

When I'm mixing these colorants with henna or cassia, I usually mix them first with water and add that mud to the henna or cassia mud. You can also mix the dried amla or indigo directly into the already prepared henna or cassia mud, adding water as needed to keep the texture smooth.

When I'm doing a two-step process of applying indigo after henna has stained hair, I make a smooth indigo pudding rather than a batter (see photo on page 107). Be sure to add enough water to make it puddinglike. If indigo is too thick, it will fall in clumps. With experience, you will find the right consistency!

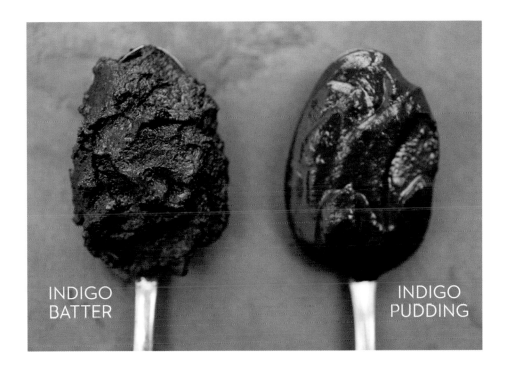

INDIGO
BATTER

INDIGO
PUDDING

Storing Herbal Colorants, Prepared and Dried

Pure herbal hair colorants are usually packaged in a sealed plastic bag inside a sturdy sealed aluminum foil package. The packages I buy weigh 100 grams, which is a little over 3½ ounces. Once opened, the herbal powders need to be stored in airtight containers to keep their potency.

Henna, amla, and cassia freeze well, keeping their ability to stain. Indigo does not keep its integrity when frozen. You may wish to store the herbal colorants differently, for convenience of use.

For henna, amla, and cassia, you can mix several batches of mud in advance and freeze them in small freezer bags, laying them flat. When you need one of the frozen mixes, pull it out from the freezer and let it thaw (usually overnight). Then simply clip the tip of a corner of the bag, and gently squeeze the thawed mud into hair. Pure henna, pure cassia, and pure amla will keep, frozen, for up to a year.

Since indigo does not freeze well, make just what you need for one application. Once opened, the bag needs to be stored in an airtight container, preferably out of the light. I always store amla and indigo in powdered form, resealing the original package and placing that inside an opaque plastic container.

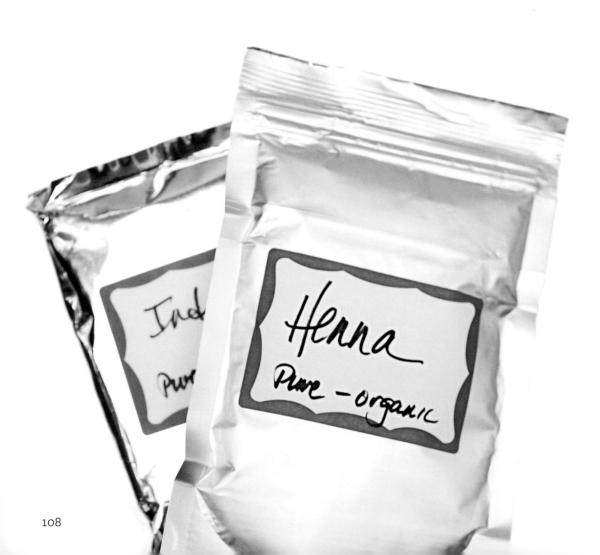

HOW TO DO A PATCH TEST

While it is true that henna, indigo, amla, and cassia are especially safe to use, the fact is anyone can be sensitive to anything. Few people experience an allergic reaction to pure henna, indigo, amla, or cassia, but if you are concerned or particularly sensitive, you can do a small patch test on your skin. Mix ¼ teaspoon of your herbal powder with a drop or two of water to form a paste. Apply the paste with your finger or a spoon to the inside of your arm or elbow crease, or the nape of the neck, close to the hairline. I prefer to test the neck because the mud can't be seen and won't be smudged off, though it is harder to see if a reaction occurs there (though you'll still be able to feel a reaction, of course). If applying to the arm, cover the mud with an adhesive bandage or some plastic wrap to keep the mud in place. Leave the herb on the skin for a couple of hours, then rinse off. (Note: If you are a professional colorist, you may want to wear a mask and gloves when using the colorants to prevent overexposure.)

Some people know when they are reacting immediately; others react after a few days or even take a few weeks to develop symptoms. You can decide when a reasonable amount of time has passed to determine if the herbal colorants are safe for you. Allergy symptoms include a tight feeling in the chest or throat, sneezing, itchy eyes, swollen eyes, swollen face, runny nose, dry cough, and hives.

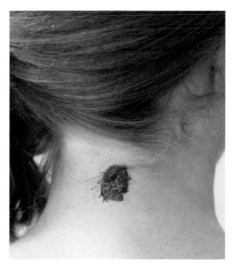

Test each color separately a few days, or better a week, apart, so you don't confuse yourself. Record your results.

Henna, indigo, and cassia may stain the skin: henna, a red tone; indigo, blue or ashy; and cassia, slightly yellow (if at all). If this happens, the stain will fade in a few hours or a few days.

THE BASIC APPLICATION PROCESS

After you've chosen your recipe and mixed your mud, it's time to get messy! Before you begin, make sure you are wearing an old sweatshirt or shirt that you don't mind staining. In my experience, it doesn't seem to matter if hair is dry or washed and somewhat wet, though I prefer to apply the mud to dry hair.

Some sources say to put cream or oil around the perimeter of your face to avoid tinting your skin, but I don't do this and have never had a problem. The dye needs to be on the skin for a good period of time to stain, plus the skin on the face near the scalp seems to be more resistant to the stain than other parts of the body. For example, I have used my bare finger to wipe fresh henna off a spoon and my finger stained immediately, yet when I'm hennaing my head and the facial area near my hairline is covered in mud for several hours, the colorant rinses right off without staining. If you accidentally get some mud on your face, just wipe it off.

Some people find it most effective to use a hair color brush or a plastic mud application bottle to apply the mud, but I prefer to use my gloved hands, as I enjoy the feeling of the mud and the fluidity of running the paste from roots to ends. If I'm using henna or indigo, I cover my hands with gloves (see box on opposite page).

STRAND-TEST FIRST?

You may wish to test your mix on a small section of hair or on hair collected from a hairbrush to see if you like the color. Just be advised that the color may look very different when it is covering your entire head. If you are up for being playful and experimental, though, and are more interested in the fun of the journey than in getting to where you want to be, then by all means, I invite you to just jump in and try it out!

Mudding the Head

When applying the mud yourself, you can section your hair and apply the mud to one section at a time, but this isn't necessary. Simply start at the crown with a good amount of herbal colorant, and work it around the head toward the face, moving from roots to ends and applying more mud as needed. Pay particular attention to the hairline around the face. The hair here is more resistant to colorants, so make sure it is covered with plenty of mud. Don't worry if you miss some spots; you'll only continue to get better. You'll be impressed with how easy it is to do after just a few applications!

TO GLOVE OR NOT TO GLOVE?

I use gloves when applying henna and indigo, not for protection against harm, but because fingernails immediately grab the stain, with henna casting a red tone and indigo a green gray. When combined with henna, indigo will turn hands black on occasion. I don't use gloves when working exclusively with pure amla and pure cassia because these colorants do not stain nails or skin, though if you are prone to sensitivities or are a professional, you may want to wear gloves when applying all herbs — too much of a good thing can challenge some bodies.

Covering the Mud

When you're done applying the mud, wrap some plastic wrap or a plastic bag around your head to keep the mud moist for better color deposit. You can put a ski cap over the plastic or wrap a scarf around your head for a striking look (see ideas for wrap styles in chapter 5). To speed up the dyeing process, you could wear a thermal cap or wrap a fresh warm towel from the dryer over the plastic to keep the mud warm. The warmth will feel especially nice over cooling henna.

Letting the Stain Set

Leave the mud on your head for at least 1 hour if using the thermal cap, or 2 hours if not. For darker colors, leave on for longer (see Playing with Staining Time on page 116). There is no limit to the amount of time you can keep these muds in your hair. Some of my clients even choose to sleep in them. While you wait, you can read, meditate, cook, do errands — whatever!

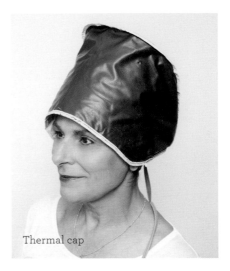

Thermal cap

Rinsing and Washing

When you're ready, remove the cap and plastic wrap. If you're using henna or indigo, the mud will be a deeper color than when you first put it on; amla and cassia muds tend to remain the same color. Now it's time to rinse.

Thus far in my experience of working with herbal pigments, cleanup is probably the least desirable part of an otherwise amazing artistic and nurturing experience. Getting the mud into the hair is fairly easy compared to getting it out. When I mud myself at home, I do a first rinse in the kitchen sink to remove the bulk of the herbal pigment, rinsing until the water runs clear. Then I jump into the shower directly after for a thorough multiwashing with shampoo and conditioner (see page 158 for product recipes and guidelines).

Safe for Drains?

One of the questions people ask me most frequently is whether the mud will cause plumbing issues at home. None of my drains at home or in my salon have been plugged from the herbal mud colorants, and I have been doing this for at least a decade!

Even with a thorough rinsing and washing, you may still find pockets of mud during the comb-out. A spritz can sometimes be enough to clean it; otherwise, it's back to the sink. Still, some women prefer to be washed and conditioned but not squeaky clean. They say that they find the color takes better if they wait until the next day to give their hair a thorough washing.

Don't be disappointed if you don't see a big color shift in your hair after it has been rinsed and shampooed. Depending on the herbal colorants, the change may be subtle or more obvious. The change is more obvious when using henna alone or in combination with other herbal colorants, though henna-indigo color combinations sometimes take a day or two after the application for the true color to unfold, so be patient. Sometimes the hair is lighter after a day or so, and sometimes it's darker.

Styling

When you're done rinsing and washing, you can dry and style your hair as you normally would. The color endures with normal care, though any color can be compromised if hair is subjected to repeated abuse.

A NEW RELATIONSHIP WITH TIME

When you use herbal hair colorants, there is no need to use a timer that dings to alert you when it's time to rush to a sink. You don't need to put up with burning eyes and scalp until it is time to wash out the color. In fact, the longer herbal hair colorants are on, as we know by now, the deeper the tone and the more lasting the stain.

While mudded, you may be doing chores, working in your garden, reading, or meditating. The beautiful thing about pure herbal colorants is that you can keep them on as long as you like, even sleeping in them should you care to.

VISUAL APPLICATION GUIDE

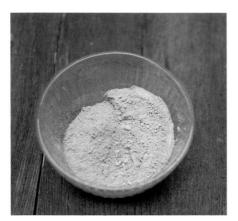

1. Start with pure powder(s), combining powders if needed.

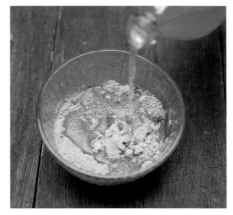

2. Add liquid to the powder (use an acid for henna and cassia and water for indigo and amla).

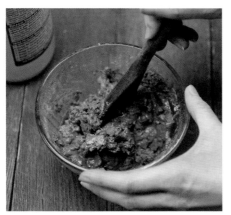

3. Mix until the colorant has a pudding consistency, adding more liquid as necessary.

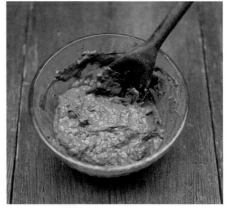

4. Let the mud sit for at least 2 hours if you're using henna or cassia.

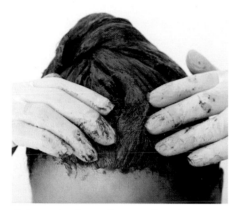

5. Apply the mud to your hair, being sure to focus on the hairline around the face.

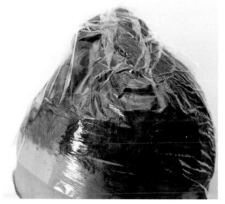

6. Wrap your head in plastic.

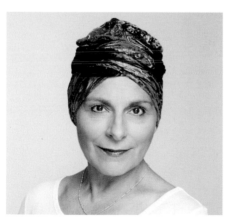

7. Wrap a scarf around the plastic (or use a thermal cap).

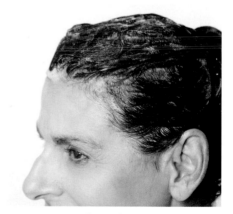

8. Rinse out the mud. Shampoo, condition, dry, and style as usual.

CLEANING OFF THE MUD

Place muddy combs and clips into a water bucket to soak until the mud "melts off," and then wash them. If you're a salon professional, also disinfect them. (These herbal colorants do have disinfectant properties, but these are not recognized by state agencies.)

You can throw the shirt you wore and your headdress into the wash along with your other laundry (I've never had a problem with cross-coloring). Any mud that falls on the sink, floor, or chair can be easily wiped off. There are times when I will find a dollop of herbal mud in some hidden spot, which makes me wonder how it ever got there. Don't worry if this happens to you. In order to stain, the pigment needs to stay moist and be on a porous surface for a good length of time, which doesn't happen when it spills on the floor.

When I say "jumping into the mud," I'm not speaking metaphorically; I mean it quite literally. Enjoy!

PLAYING WITH STAINING TIME

Understanding that the longer an herbal mud pigment is allowed to stain hair, the better the deposit and depth of color, it then stands to reason that you can adjust the staining time for a desired color result. I have experimented with varying the length of staining time for different goals and have gotten excellent results. For example:

» **If you are trying to create a soft strawberry color,** rather than a deep strawberry, leave the mud mixture on the hair for 1 hour instead of 4.

» **For deep black hair,** apply henna for 4 hours, rinse, then apply indigo also for 4 hours; then wash and condition. For a gentle black, apply henna for 1 hour, rinse, and then apply indigo for 1 hour.

» **To achieve a deep brown color,** you could try applying henna for only 30 minutes, rinse, and then use indigo for 45 minutes.

Working with Two Steps

You may choose to use a two-step process for covering gray, for blending regrowth, or to achieve a certain depth of color. You could use two different recipes, applying one, letting it stain, and then applying the second recipe, or you can apply the same recipe twice.

Basic process. For all two-step processes, the procedure is simple: Apply the first mud mixture, wrap your head in plastic and a headdress or covering, and allow the herbal colorant to stain for the desired length of time. Rinse (some people shampoo, but others find this inhibits the second mud from binding well), then apply the second round (using either the same mud mixture or a different one), wrap in plastic and a headdress or covering, and allow to stain. Then rinse, wash, and condition.

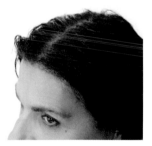 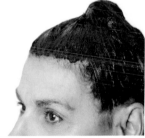 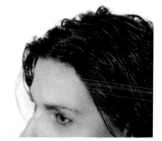

After rinsing out the first
mud mixture (henna)

Application of the second
mud (indigo)

Final rinse

Blending regrowth. It's easier to successfully blend the regrowth area when the hair is light-colored than when hair has been chemically colored a darker color and the root area is light, white, or gray, as this area will naturally grab the herbal colorants differently than the rest of the hair. If you are trying to blend a line of demarcation on brown hair, medium brown hair, or dark brown hair, and your regrowth area is significantly lighter, it can be helpful to use a two-step process. For step one, you could use henna or any combination of henna with amla, cassia, or indigo; apply the stain, rinse it out, and then apply the same combination a second time, leaving it on for an equal amount of time. Or you could use pure henna only for the first step and pure indigo only for the second step, leaving the indigo on the hair for a short amount of time — try increments of 5 minutes until you reach the desired color.

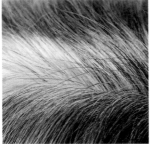 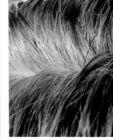 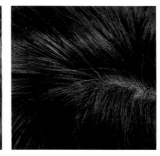

Light regrowth area | After application of henna | After application of indigo

Using indigo. I have used pure indigo for short durations to meet a variety of needs — from color corrections to blending a line of demarcation. I've achieved some beautiful coppers, reds, and browns just by using pure henna only as a "filler" first, so the grays grab better, and then using only pure indigo for various amounts of time. The same two-step approach is particularly good for virgin gray hair or gray hair that is particularly resistant to color. The first step fills the gray with pigment, which it lacks, and then the second step is for color result. Of course, part of the reason why herbal colorants are so effective and beautiful is that the more they are used, the better they work, unlike chemical colors, which produce a uniform result and can damage or dry out hair with repeated use.

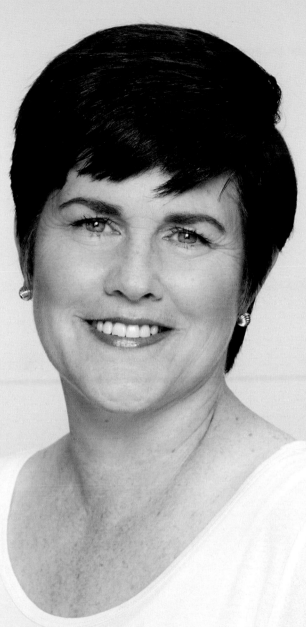

HERBAL PROCESS:
Step 1 — henna for 1 hour
Step 2 — indigo for 30 minutes

Chemical base color is medium brown with regrowth area that is 70% salt and pepper gray.

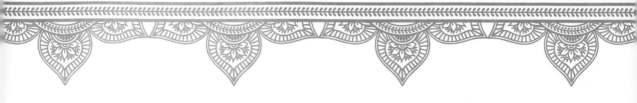

SPECIAL PROCEDURES AND CONSIDERATIONS

Herbal hair colorants should be a fun exploration. The word "exploration" indicates uncharted territory, and often there is some fear attached to the unknown because it is unknown! Approaching the unknown with enthusiasm is what our spiritual mentors encourage us to do, and while this approach might be great for our souls, it may be too scary when it comes to our hair. One purpose of this book is to equip you with enough tools, boost your confidence, and support your sense of adventure so that if something unexpected happens when you're using herbal colorants, you know what to do to get yourself to the place where you want to be.

Using Herbal Colorants on Top of Chemical Colorants

Use the same recipe and application procedure for dyeing chemically colored hair as you would for dyeing virgin hair. Sometimes the color blends perfectly with the regrowth area. If it doesn't, then you need to apply a second herbal mud colorant mix to the regrowth area. I usually start by doing a two-step of the same mix, allowing the first application to deposit color as a filler and the second to actually create the tone of the final color. If that doesn't work, then I apply pure indigo, and usually just for a short amount of time (between 2 and 30 minutes).

Assess color. It is harder to blend lighter herbal colors on dark hair than it is to blend the darker colors on lighter hair. One way to successfully blend lighter colors is to allow hair to grow a couple of inches so that you can assess the natural hair color in the regrowth area. From there, you can determine the hair's ratio of gray to natural pigment and determine, through trial and error, whether you need to use one or two applications of one particular mix or create a different mix.

Start slowly. It is wise to start with a one-step process, using one herbal color or two or more herbal colors mixed together, and assess the results. Do you like the result enough to wear it? If not, what is it that you want to change? Then apply another mud with the pigments needed for achieving your goal, and assess the color results once again. By starting with a small number of lighter colorants, you

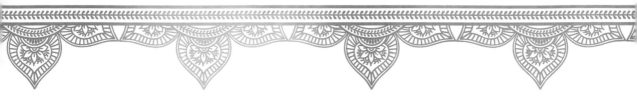

HERBAL COLORANTS AND PREGNANCY

....

Many doctors advise their patients to stop coloring their hair when pregnant. This is because chemical colorants open the hair cuticle in order to change the natural hair color in the cortex. The cortex is connected to the hair root, or papilla, and the root is connected to the bloodstream. Chemicals that are applied to the hair actually end up in the blood.

Pure, organically grown herbal hair colorants are safe to use during pregnancy. Herbal colorants stain, not damage, the cuticle. Herbal colorants that may have stained the cortex and accessed the root are not harmful. In fact, most mainstream shampoos have more questionable ingredients than pure herbal colorants. The only issue would be an allergic reaction to the herb, which is uncommon in my experience.

take the process in increments and add what is needed. It is harder to subtract what you don't want.

Mud the length of the hair. When you use herbal pigments on chemically treated hair, make sure that you bring the mud from roots to ends, especially the first several times. This will ensure that the color is blended throughout the hair shaft and that any chemically damaged hair gets conditioned. After several root-to-end applications, you can focus more on regrowth for a period; then do root-to-end applications on occasion for added color boost.

Trim it. Frequent hair trims to cut away the chemically treated color are a good practice. Eventually, the chemically colored hair will be gone.

Dyeing Virgin Gray Hair

You can use the recipes in the chart on pages 92–95 to color virgin gray hair or create your own recipe. As more gray comes in, just tweak the herbs used in the recipe or employ the two-step method.

Pure herbal dyes color gray hair differently than they color the hair's natural base color. With virgin gray hair, especially when the percentage of gray is less than the percentage of naturally occurring base hair color, the variation of color tone between the gray and the base hair color results in a highlighted effect, creating beautiful variations and a depth of color unique to the individual.

On page 124 I've shared some of my own insight and experience with how amla, cassia, henna, and indigo react with virgin gray hair. Use this information to inform your own recipe choices and tweaks.

BEFORE

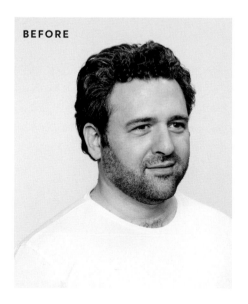

AFTER

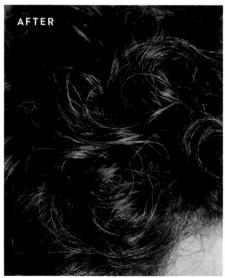

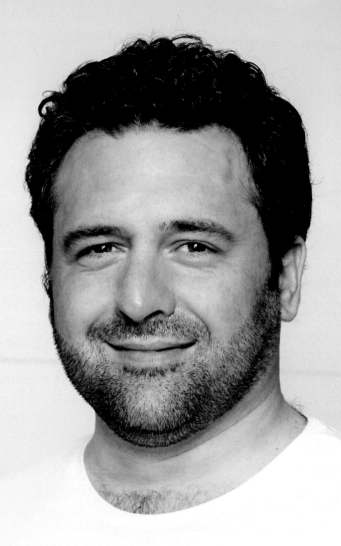

HERBAL PROCESS:
Equal parts henna and
indigo for 1 hour to check
color deposit on gray, then
reapplication of same recipe
for another hour

Base color is medium dark
brown with 15% gray, mostly
in front.

Amla. More often, I am choosing to start out using amla alone on virgin hair with 20 percent gray or less because of amla's ability to enhance hair's health. The hair shaft becomes a softer tone than the original base hair color, and color returns to gray and white hair (albeit not necessarily the original color) even though a colorant hasn't been added. Add to this amla's ability to stimulate hair growth and regrowth in thinning hair, and its general antioxidant capacity for protecting hair follicles from free radical damage and the hormones that can cause hair loss, and what's not to love?

Cassia. I like to use cassia for its soft, subtle hues of yellow and gold. After just one application of only cassia, the bright silver and white hairs are toned down, and with repeated use, cassia will take those silvers and whites to soft gold highlights. Because it deposits color gradually over time, the transition to coloring hair is not immediately noticeable. To create a quicker and slightly richer, but still almost unnoticeable, change in hair color, you could add a touch of henna (95 percent cassia and 5 percent henna). Cassia can be used to add brightness to your herbal colorant mixes and can condition bleached, damaged hair.

Henna. Herbal recipes that contain some henna are more quickly deposited, creating a more noticeable and immediate change (the abruptness of the change can be controlled by adding amla and/or cassia). Henna is less temporary than amla and cassia, so any coloring will have a regrowth area that will need touch-ups, though the regrowth area will not be as noticeable, nor will the touch-ups be as frequent, as with chemical colorants.

Indigo. Indigo is the blue/purple tone that we mix with other herbal pigments to create auburn, brown, and black. When indigo is used alone on virgin gray hair, it typically first turns hair green or teal, and then eventually purple. Your hair may also have a green tint if you are using indigo in a mix, but this too will pass. If you want to correct the green color immediately, you could apply cassia and/or henna.

HERBAL PROCESS:
60% henna, 40% indigo for 5 hours

Base color is medium brown with red undertones and 40% gray.

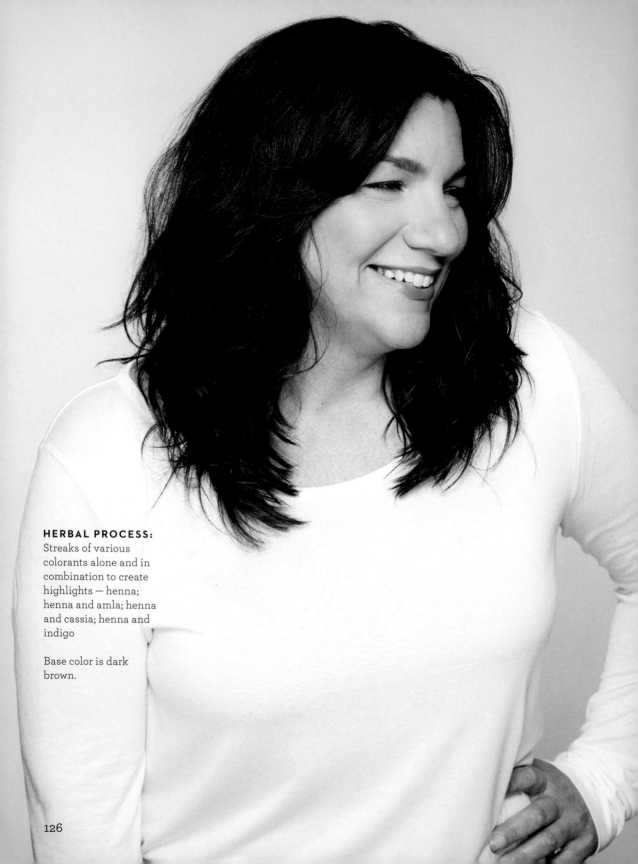

HERBAL PROCESS:
Streaks of various colorants alone and in combination to create highlights — henna; henna and amla; henna and cassia; henna and indigo

Base color is dark brown.

Highlights

Highlights are typically a chemical procedure designed to artificially replicate what sun and water do to hair in the summer. Highlights that look natural are very coveted. It is not easy to repeatedly achieve the same look with chemical colorants, because when you always highlight the same sections of hair, the already highlighted hairs usually end up becoming more and more blond, and therefore damaged. To avoid this increasingly bleached-out look when using chemical colorants, it is wise to alternate the highlight process (an accent of light colors streaked through hair) with a lowlight process (an accent of darker colors streaked through hair), or make your full head darker in the fall and winter months, then highlight once again come spring and summer.

I am often asked if I can highlight hair with plant pigments. Hair that is dyed with pure herbal pigments often has natural highlights, which are the result of how the herbal colorants deposit on the various tones of your natural base color. I can also do a "highlighting process" if the hair has never been chemically colored. The highlighting process I do is different from the one used for chemical colorants. I section hair into "chunks" and apply herbal mixtures with different tones in alternating chunks, then let the color process for at least 1 hour. Once washed and dried, the effect is quite lovely (as seen on the opposite page).

Ombré

You can achieve ombré shading with herbal colorants, though they work best for a reverse ombré look. With traditional ombré tones, hair is darker at the roots and gradually lightens toward the ends. With reverse ombré coloring, the hair is lighter at the roots and gradually darkens. Both looks require the use of more than one color to create a soft gradient effect. Reverse ombré shading can be added to any hair color — natural blond, brunette, and my favorite, natural redheads (using, of course, pure henna).

To create reverse ombré shading, section hair laterally, apply different herbal colorant mixtures to the sections, wrap, and then process.

For blond graduating to brown and black: Mix appropriate amounts of henna mud and indigo mud for your length of blond hair (keep pigments separate; see box on page 106 for quantity guidelines). Section hair laterally at the mouth level. Apply pure henna only from the mouth to the ends, and let the hair process for 1 hour or more. After rinsing, apply pure indigo only to the same section of hair and let process for 30 minutes to achieve brown. Add indigo once again to only the very bottom few inches of sectioned hair to produce black and let process for at least 1 hour. Wash and style.

For medium brown tapering to chestnut brown: Mix appropriate amounts of henna mud for your length of medium brown hair (see box on page 106 for quantity guidelines). Apply pure henna from eye level to the ends and let the hair process for 2 hours. Rinse, then apply 100 percent pure indigo from eye level to mouth level and process for 1 hour. Rinse, wash, and style.

For red tapering to black: Mix appropriate amounts of henna mud and indigo mud for your length of red hair (keep pigments separate; see box on page 106 for quantity guidelines). Section hair laterally at the mouth. Apply pure henna only from mouth level to the ends, and let the hair process for 1 hour or more. After rinsing, apply pure indigo only to the same section of hair and let process for 1 hour or more to achieve black.

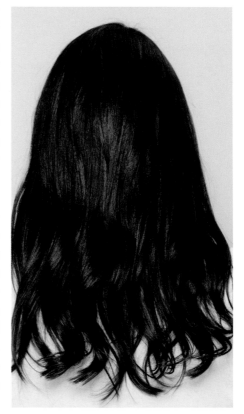

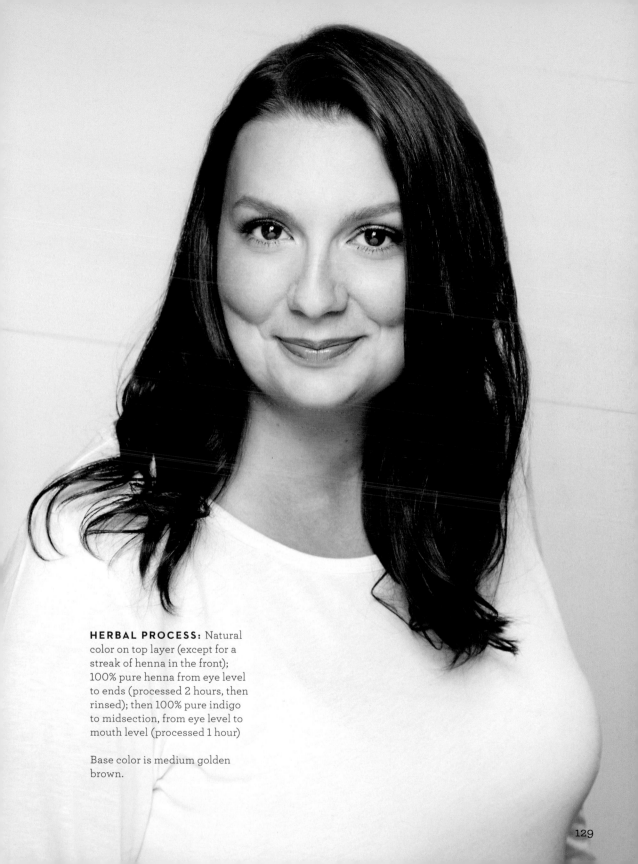

HERBAL PROCESS: Natural color on top layer (except for a streak of henna in the front); 100% pure henna from eye level to ends (processed 2 hours, then rinsed); then 100% pure indigo to midsection, from eye level to mouth level (processed 1 hour)

Base color is medium golden brown.

BASIC OMBRÉ PROCESS

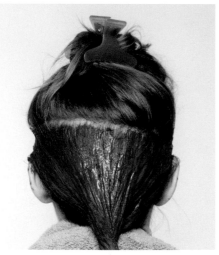

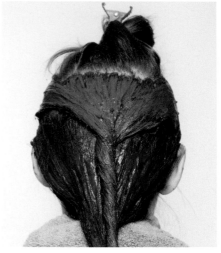

1. Section hair laterally halfway up the head and apply bottom mud.

2. Section hair at the top and apply middle mud.

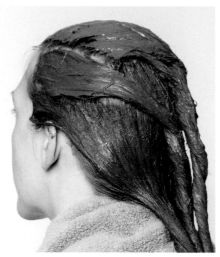

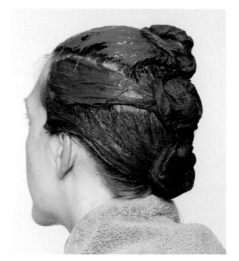

3. Apply top mud.

4. Roll mudded hair into buns and wrap with plastic and head cover. Let process for 1 hour minimum, then rinse, wash, and style.

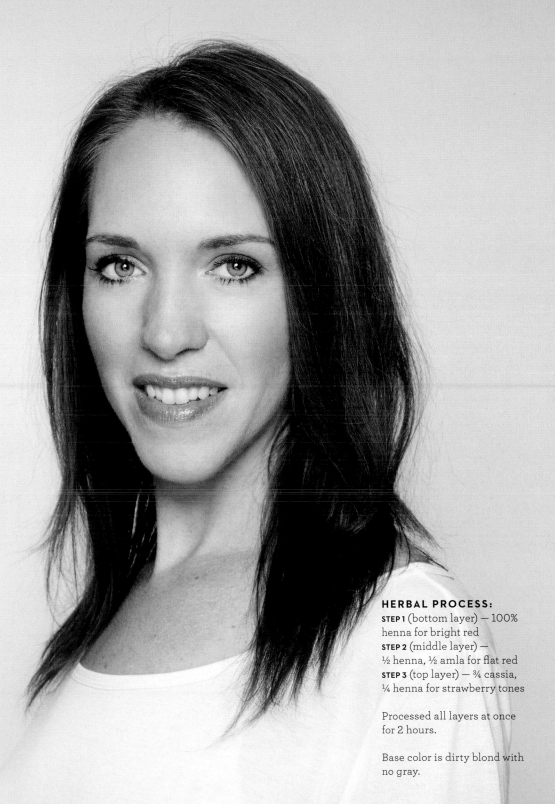

HERBAL PROCESS:
STEP 1 (bottom layer) — 100% henna for bright red
STEP 2 (middle layer) — ½ henna, ½ amla for flat red
STEP 3 (top layer) — ¾ cassia, ¼ henna for strawberry tones

Processed all layers at once for 2 hours.

Base color is dirty blond with no gray.

MAKING CORRECTIONS AND TROUBLESHOOTING

After you've applied the mud and washed and dried your hair, ask yourself if you like the result.

Need to go darker? Use more indigo in your mix, or do a quick indigo after the initial stain.

Need more red? Increase the amount of henna in the mix.

Green tint from indigo? This can happen when indigo is used on gray or white hair. The tint will usually morph overnight or wash out during the next shampoo.

Green or gray tint from ash colorants? Ash colors can be pretty and natural-looking, but if your hair doesn't take well to ash colorants, you can end up with a green or gray tint covering the desired color. If this happens, it's a sign that you should stick to warm colors in the future. In the meantime, you may add a new color in a shade that will counteract the ash tones. To determine what kind of color to use, we return to the color wheel (page 98) to understand the relationship between cool and warm colors. Ash tones have a cool, green-blue base (usually a reaction of pure indigo on gray or white hair). If we look at the color opposite green-blue on the color wheel, we find orange-red. This color will cancel out the ashy tones when

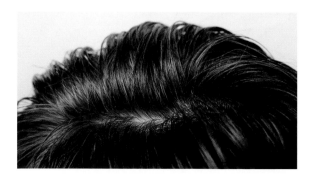

The hair is tinted green after an application of indigo over henna on white hair, but this usually disappears by the next day. See page 119 for final color.

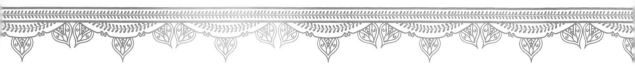

applied to the hair. Do an application of cassia, and see if this works for you. If not, you could mix and apply equal parts of henna and cassia, which should help. Henna alone may make the hair too dark.

Hair color brassy orange from henna? Hair that has too much orange is usually the result of using henna on gray or white hair. The color may tone down after a few hours. If it doesn't, you need to add a green-blue tone (again, look to the color wheel), which is created by indigo. Mix a little bit of indigo with water to create a thick liquid, and apply it to the hair for around 10 minutes. This will tone the hair to brown.

Most of the time, you can correct a color mistake. If you're still not happy with the result the second time, consider what you value most. Hair coloring has its tonal challenges no matter what the medium, and corrections are as good as the product and the experience of the one applying it, within the limits of the medium. When your expectations aren't met by reality, consider what you value — tone or texture. Some people prefer the tone be "correct," while others are less attached to color and more concerned with using natural colorants that enhance or improve hair texture and don't contain chemicals.

Remember that you don't always know how an herbal colorant will react on your hair, but as long you have an understanding of how to counter the reaction, you will find what works for you. Natural beauty is about self-discovery, so enjoy this opportunity to have some fun and solve the puzzle!

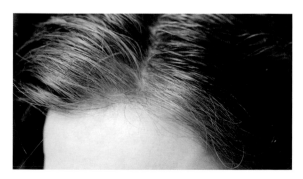

When henna is used on gray or white hair, it can produce a brassy orange. The color may tone down in a few hours. If it doesn't, simply apply indigo to this section to correct.

UNUSUAL WAYS TO USE HERBAL COLORANTS

Chunk it! One of my favorite herbal colorant procedures is to mix several different formulations, section the hair into uneven sections, and saturate each clump with a different mixture. Washed and dried, the results are stunning!

Dyed dreads. I have seen herbal colorants work particularly well on light-colored dreads, though they will work on darker-colored dreads as well. Simply saturate each dread one at a time. Dye all of the dreads the same color, or use a different color on each dread!

Rainbow crones. Make up separate batches of each of the pure herbal colorants, and apply to alternating sections of gray or white hair.

The pits. The new craze for coloring armpit hair is sweeping pits across the nation! The skin under the arms is superabsorbent and close to the breasts. While I love the idea of women embracing their pit hair, I'm just a bit concerned that repeated chemical coloring may be harmful. Why not change your coloring agent to pure herbal colorants?

Muddy beards. Yes, men muddy their beards as well as their heads! The men who come to me for coloring their beards have had reactions to chemical products made for facial hair coloring. For beards, I leave the hair unwrapped and make the herbal mud thicker so dripping isn't an issue. I let the mud process for as long as it would if it were on the head.

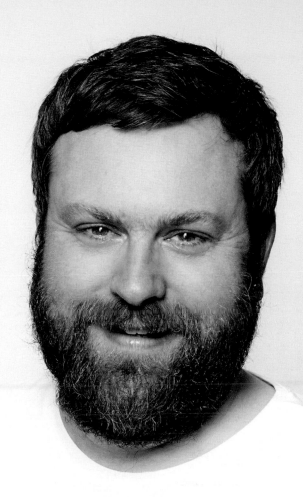

HERBAL PROCESS:
¾ cassia, ¼ henna for 1
hour

Base color is medium
gold brown.

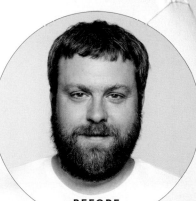

BEFORE

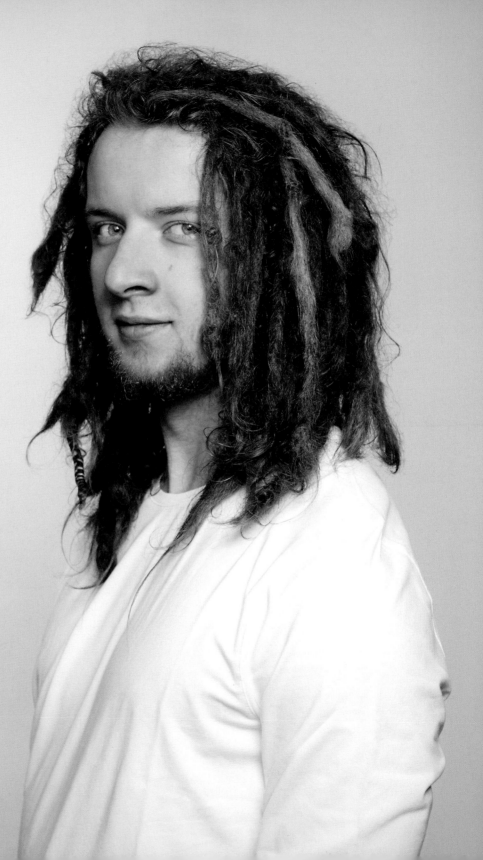

HERBAL PROCESS: Various colorants alone and in combination — henna, cassia, and indigo; henna and amla; henna and indigo; henna and cassia — processed overnight

Base color is dirty blond.

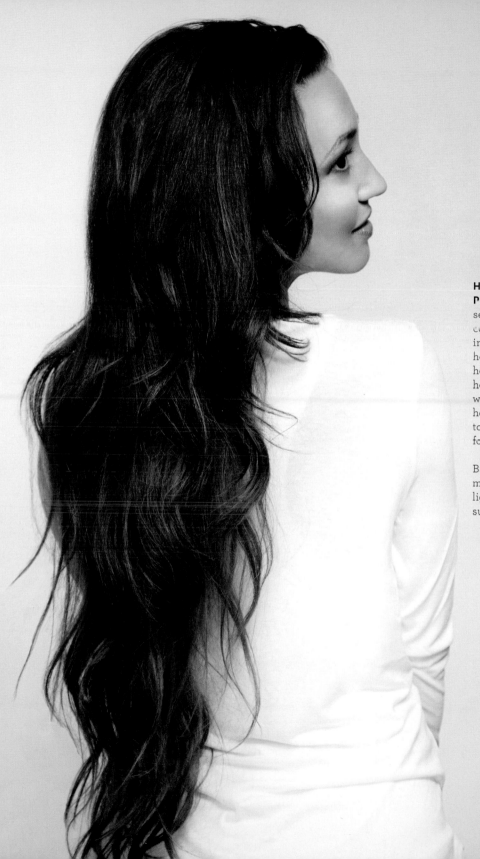

HERBAL PROCESS: Vertical sections of various colorants alone and in combination — henna and amla, henna and cassia, henna and indigo, with a few pure henna streaks toward the front — for 2 hours

Base color is a medium brown that lightens easily in the sun.

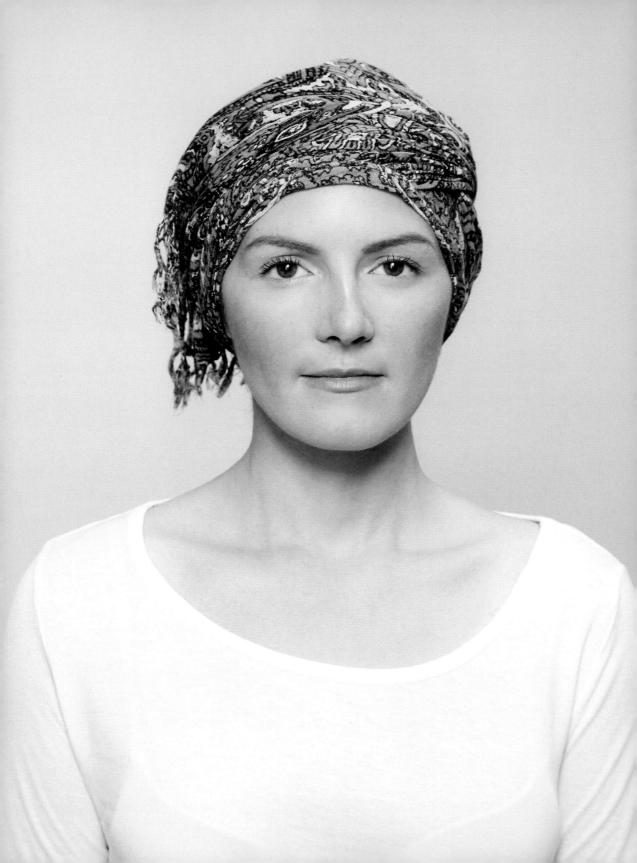

chapter five

WRAP STYLES

Beauty is a light in the heart.

KHALIL GIBRAN

Your hair is mudded with herbal pigments, and you want to leave the mud on for several hours, but you have places to go and things to do. Here are some lovely simple head coverings for your mudded mane, so that life goes on.

Embrace your goddess self! Choose among the hair wraps in this chapter for a design that suits your needs. Be sure to cover your mudded hair first with plastic to keep the pigments moist and to prevent them from staining the scarf.

When selecting a scarf, the best are those made of cotton, rayon, or acrylic. Silky scarves can slip too much. Something with a pattern will hide any minor stains that may happen from the herbal colorants.

SKULLCAPS

Skullcaps are simple, easy ways to cover mudded hair. There are many types — from cloth to knitted to the latest breathable textiles — and they can be found on numerous websites. If you knit or crochet, you most likely have made one.

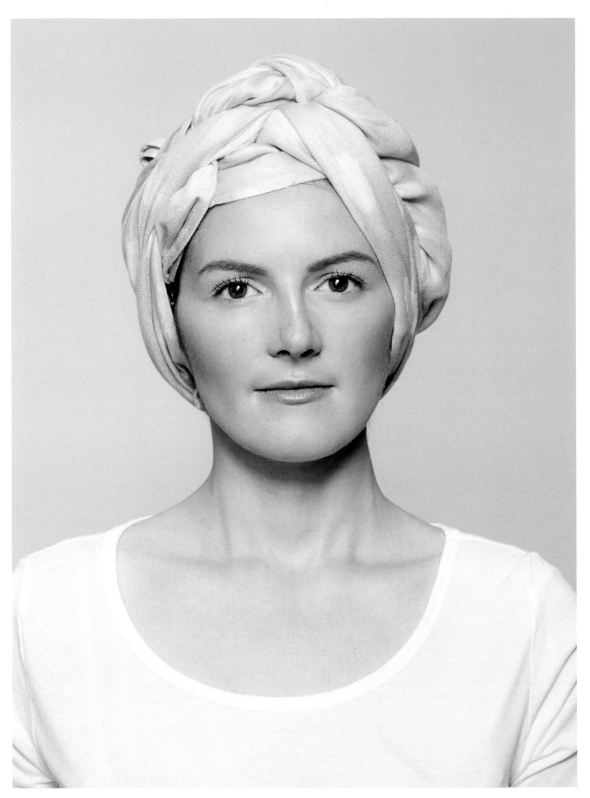

SIMPLE TURBAN

Use a large square scarf to make this turban.

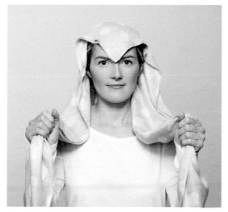

1. Fold the scarf into a triangle. Place the scarf on your head, with the triangle pointing toward the middle of your forehead and the sides hanging down toward your shoulders.

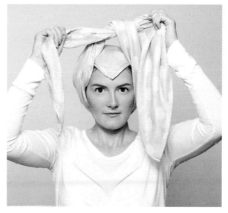

2. Bring each side to the top of your head and tie them.

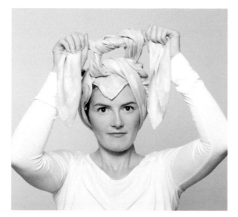

3. Tie the sides together once again to form a knot.

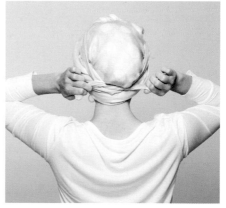

4. Bring the loose sides to the back of your head and tie them tightly together. Tuck loose ends under the front and back of the turban.

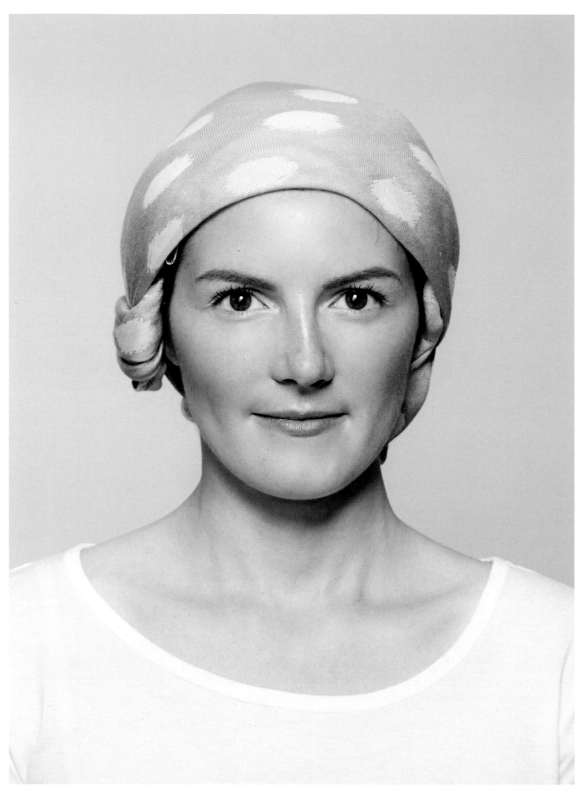

TUCK WRAP

Use a large square scarf for this wrap.

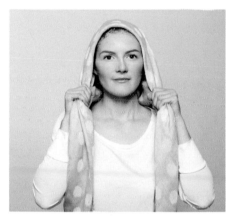

1. Fold the scarf into a triangle. Place the folded crease on top of the head, so that the fold falls along the hairline.

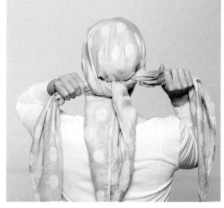

2. Hold both ends tightly, and tie the ends together at the nape of the neck. Make sure the scarf is taut and wrapped securely around the head.

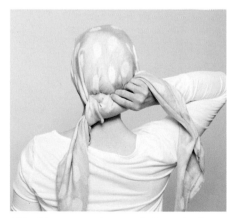

3. Tie a square knot with the ends, then roll up the center portion of cloth and tuck into the knot.

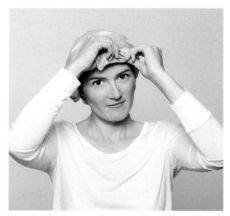

4. Tuck the loose ends into the sides of the wrap.

FAMOUS WRAPPED HEADS

I have always loved head wraps! Perhaps it's the Aries part of me that needs expression, or perhaps it's because, being five feet and one-half inch tall, I routinely need to shorten my clothes and have leftover cloth remnants that work perfectly as head bands or hair wraps. My hair also just loves being protected. I often sleep with my hair wrapped in a scarf; I find that my hair is less dry and all around happier the next morning. And I'm not alone in my love of the head wrap. For nearly a century, famous women in this country have worn the turban as a fashion statement.

Paul Poiret, a leading French fashion designer during the first two decades of the twentieth century, helped bring the turban back into fashion. Eventually, the turban was adopted by socialites such as Peggy Guggenheim and silent film stars like Gloria Swanson. In the 1930s, the turban was worn by educated, traveled women, such as the world-renowned Swedish-born film star Greta Garbo. Other notables donning head wraps include Hedy Lamarr in *Lady of the Tropics* (1939), Lana Turner in *The Postman Always Rings Twice* (1946), and Elizabeth Taylor, who accepted an award at the Sistine Chapel while wearing a head wrap (1966).

In 1996, Queen Elizabeth II wore a turban rather than crown on her tour of the Western Isles. Some current turban-wearing celebrities include June Ambrose, Salma Hayek, Kate Moss, and Sarah Jessica Parker.

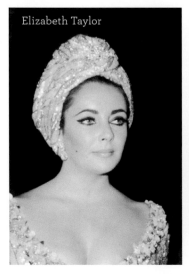

Elizabeth Taylor

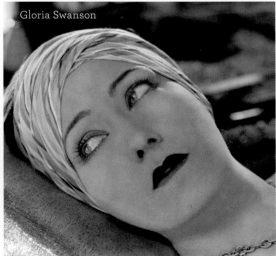

Gloria Swanson

HAIR WRAPS THROUGH HISTORY

People in most cultures have used some sort of head wrap for various reasons throughout history, and major religions — Jewish, Christian, and Muslim alike — utilize head coverings as "modest clothing" attire.

Turbans have been worn in secular cultures in Africa, Afghanistan, India, and the Middle East for as long as recorded history. Their main purpose is protection from the elements, both the blazing sun of hot climates and the freezing temperatures of cold climates. Hair wraps also help hair retain moisture, keeping hair strong and healthy.

Some of the earliest recordings of headdresses are from ancient Egypt. There, gods and goddesses were renowned for their crowns and headdresses, thus allowing people to distinguish one deity from another. Headdresses were also strongly associated with pharaohs, who wore similar crowns communicating the particular focus of a god.

In sub-Saharan Africa, the head wrap carried symbolic meaning in reference to spirituality, wealth, and social status. A woman's unique wrap expressed her individuality. In contrast, during slavery in America, certain areas of the South had legislation that required black women to bind up their hair in head wraps, serving as a marker and distinguisher of rank of female slaves. The head wrap today has taken on a message of solidarity and therefore continues to be a fashionable but conscientious statement for women of African origin.

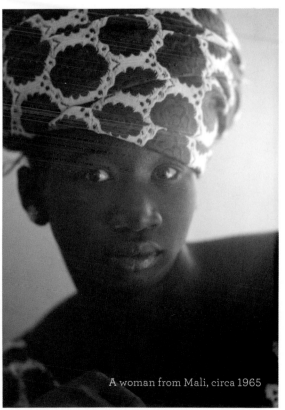

A woman from Mali, circa 1965

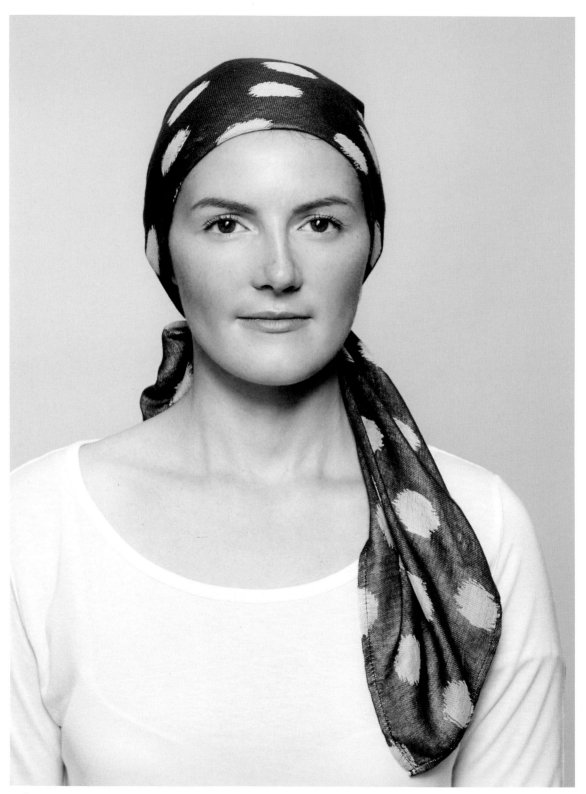

GYPSY

....

Use a square or triangular scarf to make this simple wrap.

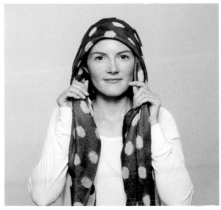

1. Fold the scarf into a triangle, and wrap it around your head, placing the folded edge along the forehead.

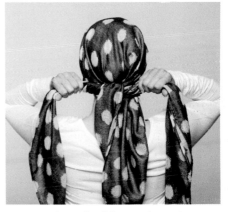

2. Tie the ends of the scarf together in the back of the head, at the nape of the neck.

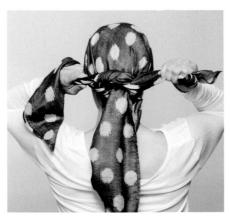

3. Tie a square knot with the ends.

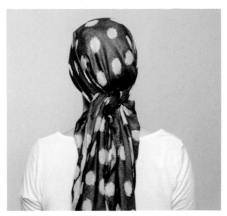

4. Let the ends hang loosely.

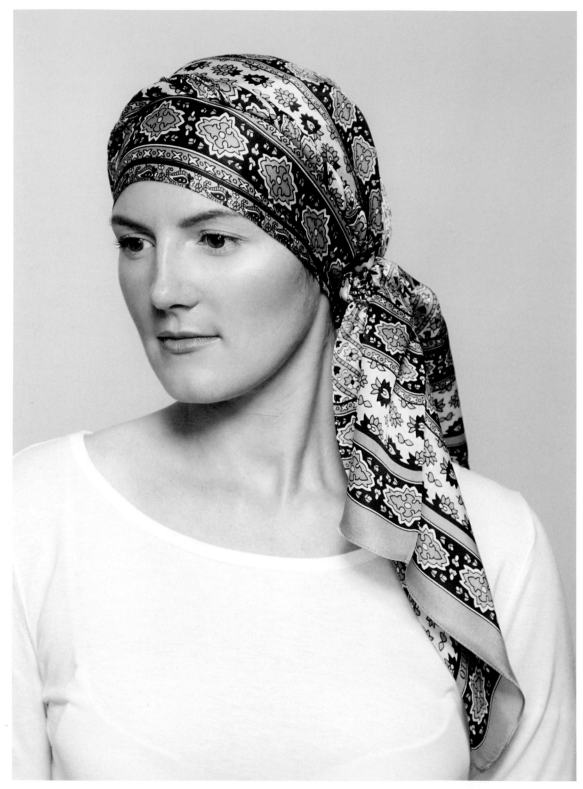

CROWN WRAP

You'll need a rectangular scarf to create this informal fabric "crown."

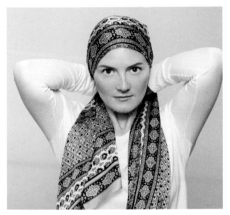

1. Drape the scarf off-center over your head, so that one end hangs lower than the other.

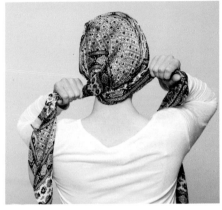

2. Bring the ends of the scarf to the nape of your neck, and cross them behind your head.

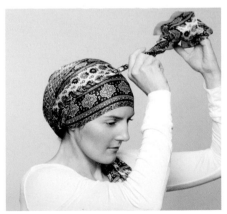

3. Twist the longer end to form a rope, and lay it on top of your head, along the front edge of the scarf (1 to 2 inches from the edge).

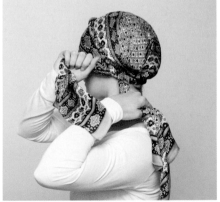

4. Run the roped end around the head, and knot the two ends together. You can leave the ends draping over your shoulder or tuck them under the back of the scarf.

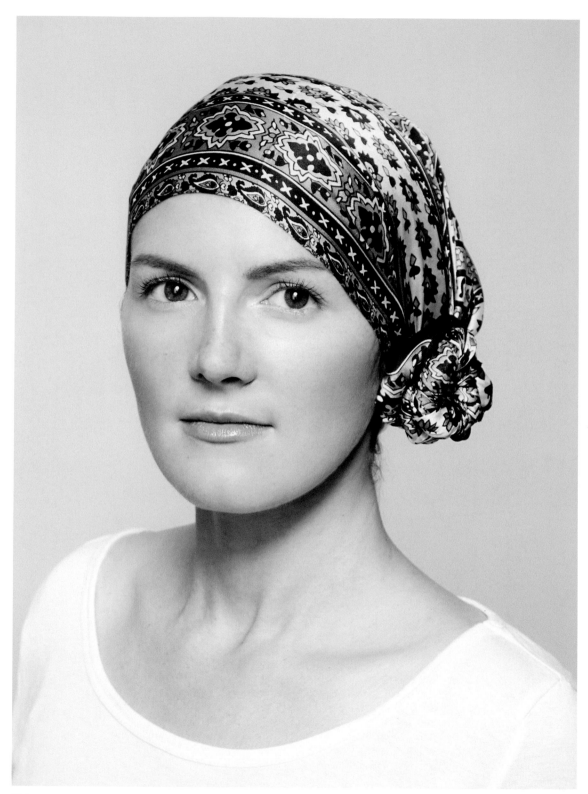

NATURAL HAIR COLORING

ROSETTE TURBAN

This turban works best with a rectangular scarf or a large square scarf with a triangle fold.

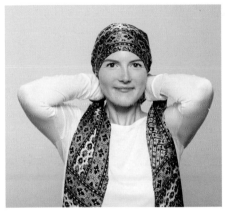

1. Place the long folded edge along your forehead.

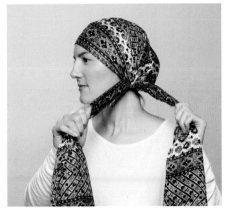

2. Bring both ends together on one side of your head and tie them in a knot.

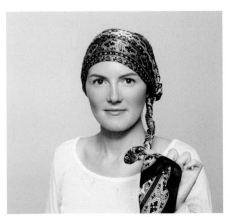

3. Twist the ends together tightly, forming a "rope," and tie in a knot at the end.

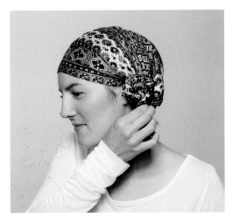

4. Circle the rope around the knot on your head, forming a rosette. Tuck the end under the rosette to secure it.

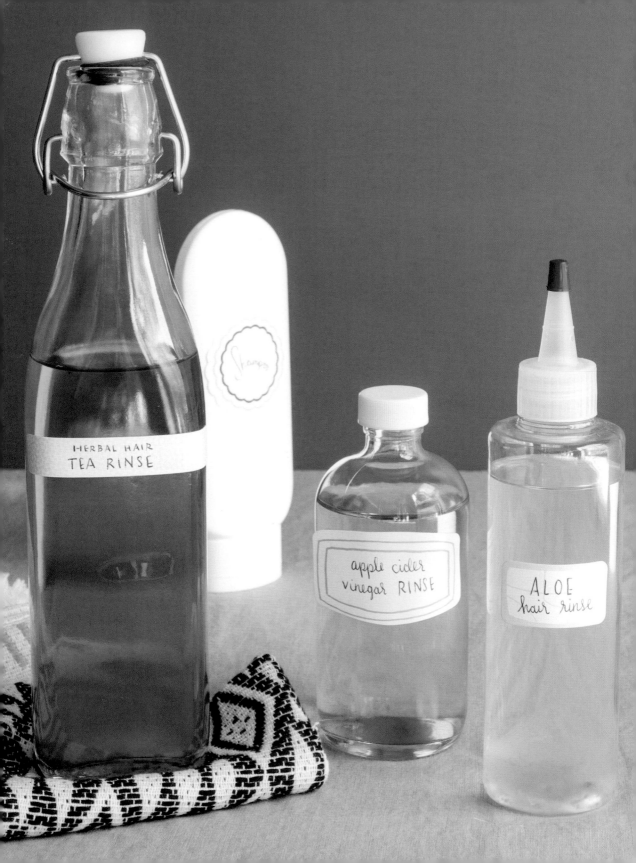

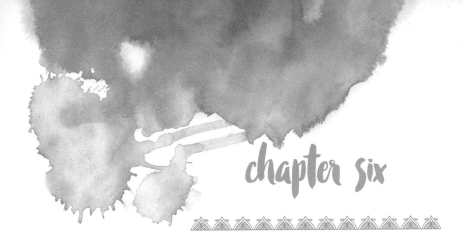

chapter six

HOW TO TAKE CARE OF HAIR
COLORED WITH HERBAL PIGMENTS

Nourishing yourself in a way that helps
you blossom in the direction
you want to go is attainable, and you
are worth the effort.

DEBORAH DAY

Herbal hair colorants hold up well no matter what type of products you use on them. Still, if you are using natural herbal pigments to color your hair, you may want to choose cleaner, safer natural and organic hair-care products for its maintenance. Here are some simple recipes using common kitchen ingredients.

HAIR CARE FOR DIFFERENT TYPES OF HAIR

Hair can be straight or curly, oily or dry, fine or coarse. Curly, dry hair has different hair-care needs than straight, fine hair. All hair types need to be treated gently, even more so when wet. Hair that is wet stretches, which allows for breakage and cuticle damage. Your activity level, exposure to the elements, and health can all affect your hair.

Assessing Your Hair Type

Humans love to place everything neatly in a box of things we "know," until one day what we know turns out to be incorrect or some new information is revealed that challenges what we know. What we know always changes. What we know now about hair types is that there are often different types of hair on one head, and there are also types within types!

There are several hair typing systems. The most common is the one developed by Andre Walker, stylist to Oprah Winfrey. His system, simplified, breaks hair into four different types. Type 1 is straight hair, Type 2 is wavy hair, Type 3 is curly hair, and Type 4 is kinky curly hair.

There is also Fia's hair typing system. This system classifies hair according to where it falls on the straight–curly spectrum, and then further defines hair by texture and overall volume, which is determined by putting the hair in a ponytail and then measuring its circumference.

BY TEXTURE

- » **Fine hair** feels like an ultra-fine strand of silk; it can also be difficult to feel a strand at all.
- » **Medium hair** feels like a cotton thread; it isn't stiff or rough, nor is it fine or coarse.
- » **Coarse hair** feels hard and wiry.

BY VOLUME

> » **Thin hair** has a ponytail circumference of less than 2 inches.
> » **Medium hair** has a ponytail circumference between 2 and 4 inches.
> » **Thick hair** has a ponytail circumference greater than 4 inches.

Care for Straight, Fine Hair

Straight, fine hair tends to be oily. It doesn't require a full application of emollient hair conditioners, but conditioners can be used on the ends of hair to reduce split ends. Straight, fine hair also has a tendency to tangle.

Fine, oily hair gets dirty much faster than coarse or thick hair. Washing hair daily can cause damage by stripping the oils the body makes for the health and upkeep of hair and skin. By stretching the amount of time between shampoos, you can allow your hair to adjust to the amount of oil it is producing. Also, instead of an emollient conditioner, you can use commercial natural hair rinses that are better for oily hair. Or try making one of the herbal tea hair rinse recipes on page 159.

Care for Curly Hair

Curly hair tends to be dry, and it is usually more fragile than straight hair. It is best to shampoo curly hair less and moisturize it more with a natural hair conditioner. On a humid day, try spritzing frequently with plain water or water that has been mixed with an essential oil.

PLASTIC COMBS CREATE ELECTRIFIED HAIR

Hair static is common in fine hair. Static happens when electrons, which are negatively charged, fly off hair, leaving hair strands with positive charges that resist each other. Plastic combs make hair static-prone, whereas wooden and metal combs do not, since these materials are conductive.

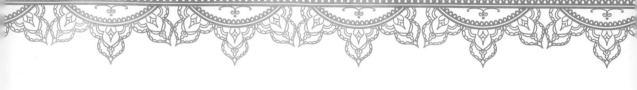

There are so many variations of curly hair that it's best I refer you to two books: *Curly Like Me* by Teri LaFlesh, which describes how people of color can take care of their curly hair, and *Curly Girl: The Handbook* by Lorraine Massey and Michele Bender, for the scoop on all curly types.

DAILY CARE FOR HEALTHY HAIR

Daily hair-care wisdom is the same for hair colored with herbal pigments as it is for any kind of hair: treat your hair kindly, meet the needs of your particular hair type, have fun with it, and if you abuse it, repair it!

Water Temperature for Healthy Hair and Scalp

While it is important to use warm or hot water when shampooing and cleaning your hair, it's generally best to use cool water when rinsing. However, the volume of hair you are rinsing matters. Because cool temperatures reduce the volume of hair, those with naturally thin hair may want to rinse with warmer water.

A NATURALLY HEALTHY SCALP

Herbal hair colorants are not only a healthy hair coloring option but also an effective remedy for scalp woes. Danduff, eczema, scalp psoriasis, and seborrheic dermatitis can disappear after a few applications.

If your scalp is itchy, it could be due to a number of reasons, from simple dandruff to an infection or an autoimmune condition. Once you determine that the cause of your itchy scalp is nonthreatening, simple home remedies such as an aloe rinse (page 162) or a vinegar rinse (page 158) can be helpful.

Cool water rinses close the hair cuticles, which helps minimize hair damage and related frizz. Closed cuticles reflect light better, and that adds shine. Cool water rinses also close scalp pores, protecting the scalp from external exposure to the elements and to hair-care products. Cool water also improves blood circulation to your scalp. As the blood moves faster, capillaries widen to warm you. With increased circulation, scalp and hair roots stay healthy, receiving the nutrients they need. Poor blood circulation reduces nutrient availability and thereby increases the risk of hair loss.

Foods That Promote Healthy Hair

Many different foods, and different diets, are good for hair. To promote hair growth, especially in today's polluted environment, any diet should contain adequate amounts of iodine. Iodine deficiency is one of the major causes of hair loss, and hair loss is one of the most common signs of an iodine deficiency. There is an abundance of foods naturally high in iodine, from seafood to potatoes; eat a balanced diet of different foods so that you're not relying heavily on one source for your iodine needs. If you decide to take an iodine supplement, take it for 3 to 4 days, stop taking it for the next 4 days, and then continue the cycle, taking it for another 3 or 4 days. This regime follows the body's natural cycle: in order to repair and heal, the body requires rest, so the 4-day break sustains the body's natural cycle of activity and rest and enhances the effects of iodine. The amount of iodine necessary for health varies from person to person; check with your doctor for what is appropriate for you.

It's common knowledge that we all need to drink enough water, but it's worth repeating. Various areas of the body are made up mostly of water. The areas of our body whose functioning is critical to our existence will receive water first when we become dehydrated; hair isn't a priority. We need to drink enough water (but not too much — excess water can flush out important nutrients) to prevent every part of our body, including our hair, from becoming dehydrated. Hair also needs water topically to maintain health.

NATURAL SHAMPOOS, CONDITIONERS, AND OTHER HAIR PRODUCTS

Anyone who knows me knows that my two favorite personal care companies are Aubrey Organics and Dr. Bronner's. Aubrey Organics products are 100 percent natural and handcrafted in the United States in batches no larger than 50 gallons, for quality control purposes. Dr. Bronner's products are also 100 percent natural, and the company has been a leader in fair trade, sustainability, and animal rights advocacy. You can use Dr. Bronner's liquid castile soap as a base to make your own homemade natural shampoo.

Simple Herbal Hair-Care Blends Made by YOU

By purchasing good-quality sustainable products, we can help create an economy that supports our values, making a larger contribution to positive change. But by making our own products from simple ingredients we most likely already have in our kitchen, we gain knowledge and empowerment, and it frees us from constant purchases. With a focus on empowerment, I share with you some of my favorite simple recipes for hair.

Apple Cider Vinegar Rinse

Raising six children naturally on a budget included homegrown food, home health remedies, and homemade personal care products. One of our favorite ingredients for all of these areas was, and continues to be, apple cider vinegar. We used it to fertilize soil, aid digestion, remedy sore throats, and rinse hair! While organic, raw apple cider vinegar from a "mother" is preferable, you can use the plain stuff from the grocery store, too.

The simplest way to use apple cider vinegar is to combine it with water and use it as a hair wash/rinse, or as a throat gargle or drink. We use one part apple cider vinegar to two parts water or herbal tea, and sometimes we add a few drops of essential oil. There is much room for flexibility.

Simple Shampoo

Mix ¼ cup water or tea (such as chamomile, hibiscus, or green tea; the list is endless, really) and ¼ cup liquid soap (I use Dr. Bronner's castile soap) in a squeeze bottle. If your hair is dry, add ½ teaspoon of olive or other oil. You can also add a few drops of your favorite essential oil if you like. Use as you would normally use a shampoo, and rinse well with cool water.

Herbal Tea Hair Rinse

My daughter Lena Moon and I loved to make herbal teas for cleaning and conditioning hair because they connect us with wildcrafting and gardening. You can use the teas as a cleanser or a rinse, and they can be alternated with store-bought shampoos and conditioners. Depending on the ingredients used, hair rinses can add moisture, cut frizz, lighten or darken hair, and more.

One tablespoon of herb per 1 cup of water is the standard measurement for an infusion (herbs steeped in hot water). The amount of rinse you need depends on how long your hair is and how frequently you will use the rinse. A good measurement to start is 2 tablespoons of herbal blend with 2 cups of water. You can keep the prepared rinse in the shower for several days, or longer if you keep it in the refrigerator.

Here are some popular herbal infusions for hair that I enjoy using:

» **DARK HAIR TEA:** sage, rosemary, black walnut hulls, nettles, raspberry leaf, and horsetail

» **LIGHT HAIR TEA:** calendula, chamomile, mullein, yarrow, and horsetail

» **RED HAIR TEA:** calendula, hibiscus, rooibos, red rose petals, rose hips, and horsetail

» **ALL-PURPOSE HAIR RINSE:** basil, fennel seed, nettle, peppermint, rosemary, sage, and horsetail

Place 2 tablespoons of your chosen herbal blend in a tea ball or muslin tea bag, or use the herbs loose and strain the infusion after steeping. Pour 2 cups of boiling water over the herbs and let steep for at least 30 minutes, covered. Remove the herbs, and let the infusion cool (remember that hair responds best to a cool water rinse, which increases blood circulation and promotes a healthy hair shaft). Add 3 tablespoons of apple cider vinegar if you wish (I like to lean my head back if vinegar has been added to ensure that it does not run into my eyes during rinsing).

Pour the infusion over your shampooed hair, massaging it into the hair and scalp. You could even "catch" the liquid in a large bowl under your head and reapply it several times. Allow the infusion to remain in the hair for several minutes, and then rinse it out, or just leave it in and towel-dry your hair. I prefer to use flour-sack cloth towels or an old T-shirt, rather than terry-cloth towels, because of their ability to absorb water but leave hair hydrated, which is especially important for hair that tends to be dry.

Sea Salt Spritz

This spritz is great for adding volume and texture to fine hair. Simply combine 4 tablespoons of sea salt and 2 cups of hot water in a medium bowl or pitcher and stir to dissolve. Pour the salt water into a spray bottle.

Wash hair in the evening; then spray with the spritz while still damp. Wrap hair in a tight topknot, and leave in the knot overnight. When you wake up the next morning, hair should be dry. Lightly spritz the topknot with the salt water; then undo the twisted hair to reveal texturized beach waves. For more texture, spray again and scrunch.

Coconut Milk Hair Mask

To add moisture to dry hair, refrigerate a can of unsweetened coconut milk overnight. Scoop the solidified coconut fat into a small bowl and save it for cooking or discard. Divide your hair into sections, and apply the milk from roots to ends,

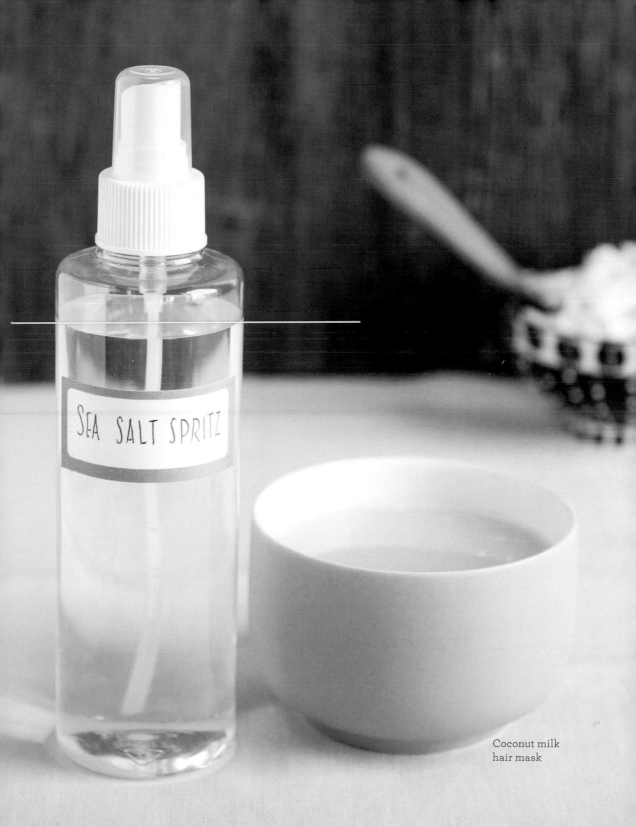

Coconut milk
hair mask

section by section, or pour directly onto your hair. Work the milk through your hair. Then place a shower cap on your head, or wrap your hair with plastic wrap, and let the mask sit for 20 minutes. Rinse your hair and finger-comb it to remove the milk mask.

Aloe Hair Rinse

To give hair texture and definition (good for hard-to-control hair), you can try an aloe hair rinse to make the hair slightly stiff. Mix one part pure aloe vera juice with two parts water in a pitcher or squeeze bottle. Shampoo the hair; then rinse with the aloe mixture. If you prefer hair that is less stiff, use less aloe, or rinse the hair with plain water after using the aloe rinse.

Vegan Hair Gel

To get started with this easy recipe for homemade hair gel, combine ¼ cup whole flaxseeds and 2 cups water or herbal tea in a small saucepan. Bring to a boil; then reduce the heat and simmer, stirring constantly, for 20 minutes, or until the mixture gels. Strain the gel into a jar. The hair gel will keep for up to 1 month in the refrigerator.

Gelatin Hair Gel

To make a gelatin hair gel, pour 1 cup of boiling water or herbal tea into a medium bowl. Stir in gelatin. For a soft hold, use ½ teaspoon gelatin; for a medium hold, use ³/₄ teaspoon; for a firm hold, use 1 teaspoon. Make sure the gelatin is completely dissolved. Refrigerate or allow to sit out until cool (especially if you're putting it in a plastic squirt bottle for use). Add a drop or two of essential oil if you like.

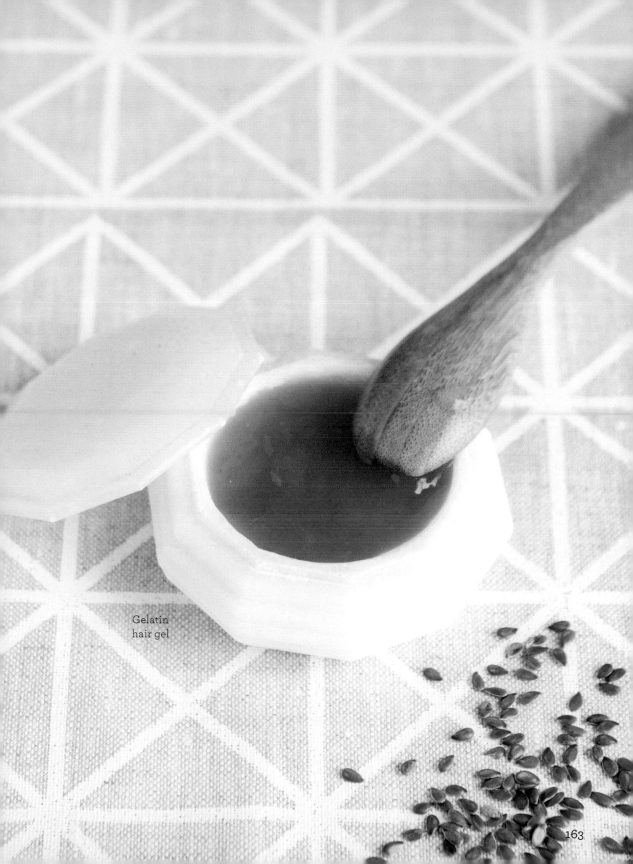

Gelatin
hair gel

How to Choose the Right Product

Shopping for natural products can be overwhelming, since there is no standard for what is "natural." Beautiful packaging and "buzz" words create a "hook" on the front of the box, though it's the ingredients on the back that count most when you know that up to 60 percent of topical ingredients are absorbed directly into the bloodstream within 20 seconds of your lathering on the product. Being an informed shopper takes time, but it is well worth the effort.

There are copious amounts of personal care products in the marketplace all vying for your attention. It can be challenging to find an authentic organic beauty care product. Labels can be hard to read, using unfamiliar language, or ingredients may not be "fully disclosed." Don't hesitate to call and ask for a full-disclosure ingredient list. If you are committed to finding natural or organic personal care products, you need to know what you are looking for.

Labeling standards. Manufacturers must use ingredient identification standards, and many use labels that adhere to the International Nomenclature of Cosmetic Ingredients (INCI) system. Honorable companies use the INCI name with the common name in parentheses — for instance, *Mangifera indica* (mango) seed butter. Or they use their own symbol system to explain more details.

Organic ingredients. These are usually noted with a star (*). I like to see that at least 70 percent of a product's active ingredients are organic and stars are plentiful.

What's at the top of the list. Ingredients must be listed in order of concentration by weight. The first ingredient is what there is the most of in the product, with the remaining ingredients listed in descending order of concentration.

Where there is water, there is preservative. Lotions, creams, moisturizers, and foundations all contain water and oil. To blend together, they need to be emulsified (suspending a liquid in another liquid). Whenever you are using liquids (water, juice, tea, aloe), you need to use preservatives to inhibit bacterial growth. While

FIVE-STEP GREEN SHOPPERS GUIDE

Before leaving my former employer to start Faces of Astarte, I created a simple five-step green shoppers guide (though we implemented only to step four) to enable people to see at a glance how "clean" or eco-friendly their favorite products were, and which products could use some improvement. You might wish to implement something similar for the products you find.

Step 1. Products are mostly synthetic or sourced from fossil fuel, with some natural or organic ingredients. These products are often found in grocery stores or corner pharmacy stores.

Step 2. Products are mostly natural or organic, with fewer petrochemicals and chemical preservatives.

Step 3. Products are "all natural" without certifications (which are very expensive). Smaller local companies are the main providers of these products.

Step 4. Products are 100 percent natural with certifications.

Step 5. Products are 100 percent natural with certifications, plus they come from a company that adheres to sustainable practices, pays employees a living wage, and uses eco-friendly packaging (i.e., it's not just recyclable but made from recycled and/or biodegradable materials).

the percentage of water and oil may be high compared to the percentage of active ingredients, as a whole, antioxidants, enzymes, peptides, and vitamins are effective in small amounts. This is why infusions or decoctions are still very effective, while less demanding on the ecosystem than concentrated essential oils. Some innovative natural companies have patented their own 100 percent natural preservatives and methods, so look for those.

Fragrance and parfum. These are considered trade secrets by the FDA, so precise formulas do not have to be disclosed on the label. You may be able to tell, however, if they are naturally derived or essential oil blends. A "fragrance" or "parfum" on the label can also indicate an artificial fragrance, which can be an irritant for those with sensitivities. High dosages of even natural essential oils can also be irritating to those who are sensitive.

You don't always get what you pay for. Some of the purest and most effective products are also reasonably priced. "Best" does not necessarily equate with "expensive." Sometimes it's best to shop for the manufacturer who fits your values down the line. Some manufacturers will make a few pure products and then we assume their whole line is pure, though this may not be true. Some manufacturers will make products that run the gamut from pure, natural, and organic to nothing pure, natural, or organic. Find a company with a passion for making a difference in why they make what they do and how they do it, and you will always be satisfied.

All certifications are not the same. While this does mean more engagement on your part to know which certifications mean what, the USDA and Soil Association certifications require that 70 percent of non-liquid ingredients must to be grown, harvested, and extracted organically.

What is this ingredient? The Skin Deep Cosmetics Database by the Environmental Working Group (EWG) is one good way of getting the scoop on your favorite products (go to ewg.org, then Skin Deep). Plug in an ingredient or product, and EWG scores the product or ingredient using a scale from 0 to 10. A score from 0 to 2 means low hazard, 3 to 6 means moderate hazard, and 7 to 10 means high hazard.

Because there are no requirements for health studies or pre-market testing of the chemicals in personal care products in the United States, part of EWG's mission is to disseminate known data and get the FDA to make sure all ingredients are tested before they are used in public formulations. Because of this, safe products sometime get a higher hazard score even if their ingredients are 100 percent plant-derived, due to lack of data.

I also encourage you to do individual ingredient searches online, where there are many options for information, including a material safety data sheet (MSDS), which is a report containing information on potential hazards (health, fire, reactivity, and environment) and safe use of various substances.

Once you get the hang of it, finding products that fit your values will come easily.

HAIR STYLING

All hair types benefit from air drying, though many of us use heat to style our hair directly after washing. Over the long term, repeated exposure to heat causes bubbles to form in the hair shaft, making it brittle and easily breakable. If you have to use a hair dryer, use sparingly and when possible use low heat settings to prevent serious damage.

You can style hair colored with herbal colorants just as you would style untreated hair. It's safe to use any type of styling device, such as curling and straightening irons, though these can dry out even oily hair if they're used too much. Don't use styling devices on wet hair or on high settings, and give your hair a break from styling from time to time so it doesn't break!

You can style hair colored with
herbal colorants just as you would style
untreated hair.

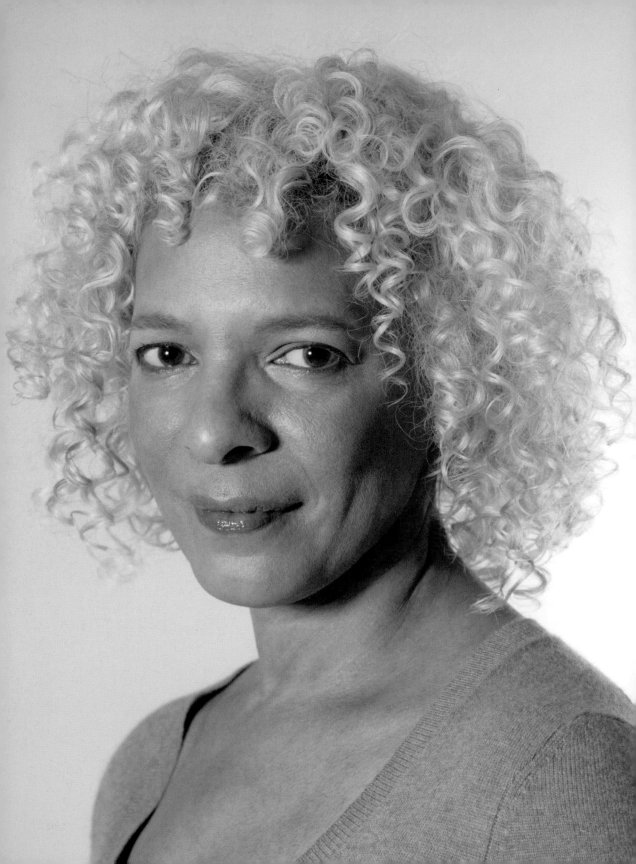

chapter seven

FREQUENTLY ASKED QUESTIONS

You can take no credit for beauty at sixteen. But if you are beautiful at sixty, it will be your soul's own doing.

MARIE STOPES

Do herbal colorants work on 100 percent gray or white hair?

Yes. Herbal colorants will cover 100 percent gray and white hair, though remember that when using the chart on pages 92–95 or formulating your own recipe, gray or white is your natural base color. Sometimes the processing time is longer for 100 percent gray or white hair. Some hair requires at least 6 hours for good coverage.

Should I test the herbal colorants on my skin or my hair before I try them?

Yes. While it is true that henna, indigo, amla, and cassia are especially safe to use, anyone can be sensitive to anything. Allergy symptoms include a tight feeling in the chest or throat, sneezing, itchy eyes, swollen eyes, swollen face, runny nose, dry cough, and hives. If you experience any of these symptoms after testing the herb, do not use it. See page 109 for instructions on how to do a patch test.

Do herbal colorants and perms go together?

You can mix herbal colorants and perms, and there are less toxic, gentler perms available. I find that it is best to do the perm before you do the color. Ask your stylist to use a smaller rod for a tighter curl because herbal colorants, particularly henna, soften curls — possibly due to the added weight of the stain on the hair shaft.

Can I use chemical colors or bleach on hair that has been dyed with these herbal colorants?

Yes, depending on the chemical product. I have successfully used a chemical colorant that is ammonia-free with a low level of hydrogen peroxide and no more than 2 percent PPD over herbal hair colorants. A mild bleach formula can lighten a too-dark henna or indigo dye, though the bleach can turn the color brassy.

Can I use the herbal colorants over a chemical tint?

Yes! Herbal colorants can and are successfully being used over chemically treated hair.

How can I remove herbal stains from my hair?

You have several options. You could wash your hair more frequently, using a peppermint liquid castile soap; you could use an ammonia-free, low-peroxide chemical colorant with 2 percent PPD over the herbal colorant; or you could grow your hair out, as the color will continue to wash out and fade over time.

Can I lighten my hair after using henna or indigo?

You can use a hair lightener or mild bleach to lighten a too-dark henna or indigo dye, though the bleach can turn the color brassy.

How often can I use herbal colorants?

If you use pure powered herbal colorants, there is no limit to the frequency with which you can apply them. You could feasibly apply the mud daily for a period of time to achieve a particular depth of color (it's just a lot of work, and the change is gradual). There is also no time limit for keeping these colorant muds in your hair. Indigenous people who live where these plants are grown often sleep with the muds on to get deeper, longer-lasting color results.

Will the herbal mud clog my drains?

None of my drains at home or in my salon have been plugged from the herbal mud colorants, and I have been doing this for more than a decade!

Will heat affect the staining process?

You can speed up the staining process by using heat, in the form of either a warm towel wrapped around your head or a thermal cap (see page 112).

What do I do if I get some herbal mud in my eyes?

It's not common to get herbal colorants in the eye, but if you somehow manage to do that, flush the eye with cool water as you would for any irritant.

Will the herbal muds stain my floor, chair, or counter, if some accidentally spills?

Henna could stain a porous surface in a short amount of time, though it's highly unlikely that it will stain any finished surface. Indigo and cassia take much longer to stain a surface; you likely would have cleaned up the muds before they have a chance to stain.

How often should I shampoo my hair after mudding?

There are no special washing instructions particular to herbal colorants. Wash your hair according to your hair type (see page 154).

How long will the stain last on my hair?

The color can shift in tone a few days after mudding, settling into one tone at that point. Remember that, while semi-permanent, these pigments will fade somewhat near the regrowth area. Regrowth touch-ups are generally done between 4 and 8 weeks, depending on how fast your hair grows.

Is it possible to apply the herbal muds too frequently?

Perhaps if you are predisposed to a sensitivity, you might discover the sensitivity more quickly from more frequent applications. But if the herbal pigments are pure and you don't mind doing the colorants more often, there shouldn't be an adverse issue for your hair.

Will my hair smell like the herbal mud after I've washed and dried it?

Some people say they smell the mud for a week, some say the smell disappears when they wash their hair, and others say they don't smell it at all. Perhaps it depends on the sensitivity of your nose!

Are herbal muds safe for children?

Yes, herbal mud colorants are safe for children. Several of my clients who are moms bring in their daughters for henna treatments without issue. Again, anyone can have an allergy to anything.

How do I know if I have a pure herbal product?

Before you purchase a product, there are a few things to watch for: The herbal colorant should only come in powdered form; if it comes in a cream, block, or paste, it has additives of some sort. If the directions say to use boiling water, it's possible that the colorant contains metallic salts, which are released by the boiling water. And if the directions say the stain will happen quickly (in less than 1 hour), the colorant is probably not pure. Once you've purchased a product, there are also a few tests that you can run. See page 66 for instructions on how to test henna for purity and page 73 for how to test indigo.

Are the herbal powders used for coloring hair edible?

If the herbal powders are pure, they can be ingested. Some, particularly amla, have many health benefits. As with any herb or supplement, however, talk to your doctor before consuming.

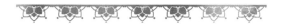

IN CLOSING

That which is striking and beautiful is not always good, but that which is good is always beautiful.

NINON DE L'ENCLOS

It is very important that consumers realize that while labels today make all kinds of claims on the front, it is the back label with the fine print that they need to pay attention to. Remember: Companies use their labels for marketing purposes (referred to as "real estate") as well as information. We each must be engaged enough to read the labels rather than basing our purchase decisions on marketing claims or recommendations from store staff — whether at conventional stores or natural food stores. There are so many products at the big "natural products" trade shows that are not natural, and many times big conventional companies buy up cutting-edge natural lines; it's hard for staff to be on top of all that "stuff."

Since there are currently no governmental standards for organic personal care products, you are left to set your own standards, and label reading is the tool for checking whether a product meets them. By taking charge, you will learn not only about the products but also about the companies. Some companies may sell only products that are 100 percent natural, while others may have some products that are 100 percent natural as well as other products that are 0 percent natural. I prefer to support companies with a commitment to a natural, organic lifestyle across the board.

In your quest, you may run into a couple of common stumbling blocks. Many big-name brands will feature a few "organic" ingredients on the front of their label, but when you look on the back you will see the rest of the ingredients are not natural or organic (the words "natural" and "organic" are *not* synonymous). You might also believe that natural products are more difficult to use because they are different, but different does not equate to difficult. Once you understand how they work, there is no issue. We have been taught not to think about how to use a product but to follow directions. With natural products, there is more room for "play" and experimentation. There is more learning about who you are as an individual and what works or doesn't work for you.

Being an avid label reader gave me an intimate understanding of natural products and products in general, allowing me to create the cutting-edge natural health and beauty department at a premier natural foods store. Before leaving there to create my salon and spa, I created the Five-Step Green Shoppers Guide (page 165) that is on display at that store to this day. This guide gives consumers a quick shopping reference.

Technologies change, and because of these changes, how we live changes as well. Take for example the industrial revolution. It changed lives, improved the health of the economy and of families, and served as an important part of our shared story. As with any construct, it worked for a time until it no longer did; at some point, what works with positive impact has the reverse effect — where it once helped, it now hinders or hurts. When what once worked no longer does, we can no longer ignore change; our choice becomes whether we resist or accept it. This is true for everything, including personal relationships.

The time of change is a time of transition, and if you have ever birthed a child, you will know that transition is the most intense time of the birthing process. It happens just before the goal is attained — in this case, the baby's arrival. Some women are able to harness the raw energy and transmute it from pain to pleasure, while others need to just get through it; in either case, the result happens anyway.

Our struggling economy, which has been sluggish for nearly a decade, is actually an indication of the current transition we are in. A transitional economy arises when the past is passing and the future has not quite arrived, and its presence is revealed by how people are spending their very hard-earned money. Because their money is hard-earned, informed and caring consumers have decided that the easiest way to create change is to back fiscally what they want to create. They are voting with their currency to support what they value — other people's labor and lives; a clean, healthy, sustainable environment; and a robust economy.

Looking forward now, I understand that my journey is your journey. A passion for natural products and an experience with environmental activism have combined in my heart and psyche. Faces of Astarte is more than just a place to get natural beauty services and products. It is a place of renewal, of re-envisioning who and what we are, what beauty is and can become. My life has been a mission to support individuals' efforts to build community and keep our resources safe, one person at a time in my chair.

This purpose-inspired journey continues beyond this book. I am offering an in-house internship program for those seeking direct hands-on learning, as well as online classes.

It is wonderful to witness our collective growth, where we intentionally make space in our lives, individual purchases, and communication to support a transition to an economy based not on exploitation of resources and others but on care, collaboration, and conservation. When you come to me looking at products for yourself, and you ask me, Is this organic? Is this cruelty-free? Fair trade? I witness the result of personal steps taken decades ago, and I am excited and inspired!

We've reached a place in our current beauty culture where what we've been doing, though beneficial in the past, is not working anymore. We need to grow and morph. Deciding how beauty is quantified, and what it means to be a unique beauty, is integral to the success and happiness of the next generation of consumers and service providers. These are exciting times! As Nahko of Medicine for the People sings, "We're a part of something special" and "I believe in the good things coming."

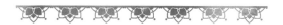

GLOSSARY

base color. This is the current color of your hair, whether it's your natural color or the color from chemical or herbal dyes. Your base color is the color you take into account when formulating your herbal colorant recipe to produce a specific hair color.

chemical colorant. A synthetic, man-made color, distinct from plant or herbal pigments.

cortex. The cortex constitutes the bulk of the hair fiber. It is made up largely of keratins, a family of proteins that also provide the tough outer sheath of skin cells.

cuticle. This is the armor of the hair shaft. Made up of thin scales of dense keratin, it protects the cortex from physical and chemical damage. When the cuticle is damaged by chemicals or physical trauma, the cortex is exposed and open to damage. The visible result of such damage is broken hair and split ends.

decoction. A method of extracting oils and volatile organic compounds from herbs by boiling. Herbs are added to water and brought to a boil, then simmered, then steeped for a time.

follicle. Within the hair follicle is the onion-shaped hair bulb in which the hair root is connected to the body's blood supply via the papilla. Nutrients produced in the lower part of the bulb are converted into new hair cells, and as they grow and develop, these cells steadily push the previously formed cells upward, creating "growth" of the hair shaft.

herbal mud. Refers to herbal powders that have been mixed with a liquid (water, acid, or herbal tea) to produce a "mud" paste/batter that is applied to hair to color it.

infusion. A method of extracting flavors and volatile organic compounds from herbs by pouring boiling water over them and allowing them to steep for a time.

medulla. A central core of round cells found in the hair's cortex.

melanin. This the pigment the gives color to skin and hair.

papilla. The part of the hair root that is connected to the body's blood supply.

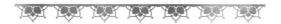

RESOURCES

SOURCES FOR PURE HERBAL COLORANTS

There are many great sources for pure herbal colorants. Remember that pure does not mean non-allergenic. I source my own line using a reputable company that complies with the certifications I value:

GODDESS BEAUTY, LLC
Little Falls, New York
315-868-7960
www.christineshahin.com

Other places to purchase pure plant pigments:

ARTISTIC ADORNMENT
Boston, Massachusetts
617-429-6301
www.artisticadornment.com

HENNA CANADA
705-444-6861
http://hennacanada.ca

HENNA CARAVAN
Camarillo, California
800-894-3662
http://hennacaravan.com

HENNA FOR HAIR
Kent, Ohio
855-634-2634
http://hennaforhair.com

HENNA MOON
Exmouth, Western Australia
info@hennamoon.com.au
www.hennamoon.com.au

HENNA SOOQ
Elkridge, Maryland
410-579-4543
www.hennasooq.com

RENAISSANCE HENNA
London, United Kingdom
www.renaissancehenna.com

And some sources for other herbs:

CHAGRIN VALLEY SOAP & SALVE COMPANY
Solon, Ohio
440-248-7627
www.chagrinvalleysoapandsalve.com

FRONTIER NATURAL PRODUCTS CO-OP
Norway, Iowa
800-669-3275
www.frontiercoop.com

MOUNTAIN ROSE HERBS
Eugene, Oregon
800-879-3337
www.mountainroseherbs.com

STARWEST BOTANICALS
Sacramento, California
800-800-4372
www.starwest-botanicals.com

RECOMMENDED READING

Falconi, Dina. *Earthly Bodies & Heavenly Hair.* Ceres Press, 1998.

Hampton, Aubrey. *Natural Organic Hair and Skin Care*, 2nd ed. Organica Press, 1990.

Janssen, Mary Beth. *Pleasure Healing.* New Harbinger Publications, 2009.

Kreamer, Anne. *Going Gray.* Little, Brown and Co., 2007.

McCain, Marian Van Eyk. *Elderwoman: Reap the Wisdom, Feel the Power, Embrace the Joy.* Findhorn Press, 2002.

Miczak, Marie Anakee. *Henna's Secret History.* Writer's Club Press, 2001.

Northrup, Christiane. *Goddesses Never Age.* Hay House, 2015.

Walker, Andre. *Andre Talks Hair!* Simon & Schuster, 1997.

Weinberg, Norma Pasekoff. *Henna from Head to Toe!* Storey Books, 1999.

RECOMMENDED WEBSITES

BLACK GIRL WITH LONG HAIR
http://blackgirllonghair.com

CONSCIOUS AGING ALLIANCE
Sage-ing International
http://sage-ing.org/the-conscious-aging-alliance

DR. BRONNER'S
www.drbronner.com

HENNA CARAVAN
www.hennacaravan.com

THE HENNA PAGE
www.hennapage.com

HERBS TREAT AND TASTE
http://herbs-treatandtaste.blogspot.com

I AM A SUCCESS STORY
www.facebook.com/IAmASuccessStory/

INDIANA HEMOPHILIA & THROMBOSIS CENTER, INC.
www.ihtc.org
Information on G6PD

MEDICINAL HERB INFO
http://medicinalherbinfo.org
Information on indigo

NATIONAL ASSOCIATION OF ECO-FRIENDLY SALONS & SPAS
www.naefss.org

NATURALLYCURLY.COM
www.naturallycurly.com

RED TENT TEMPLE MOVEMENT
http://redtenttemplemovement.com

REGISTRAR CORP.
www.registrarcorp.com

SAGE-ING INTERNATIONAL
http://sage-ing.org

TIGHTLY CURLY
www.tightlycurly.com

UNITED STATES DEPARTMENT OF AGRICULTURE
www.usda.gov

WOAD IS ME
University of California, Los Angeles
www.botgard.ucla.edu/html/botanytextbooks/economicbotany/Isatis

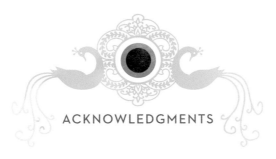

ACKNOWLEDGMENTS

When we try to pick out anything by itself, we find it hitched to everything else in the universe.

JOHN MUIR

For such a simple book, the souls to which I am deeply grateful are many. In naming the names, I hope not to overlook anyone or seemingly elevate some over others. To those not listed here — I love you and I am grateful for you.

TO MY BELOVEDS

Steven Albert Wood, who knows firsthand what it is like to live with an impassioned, narrowly focused paradigm shifter; thank you for walking this journey next to me as friend, father and birthing partner of our brood, creator of family and music extraordinaire, husband, and bestower of unconditional love and forgiveness.

The Brood: Jamie Dubois, Steven Albert Jr., Lena Moon, Radney Hamilton (The Rad Pastor), Christopher Bronson (C), Trevor Colin (Guy), and Shadia Fayne. You each inspire me always in all ways to become the best I am capable of being, especially when I doubt it myself. Thank you for receiving and returning our love.

Fr. Michael Shahin (Daddy), thank you for teaching me that faith is dynamic and to be lived and how to accept with dignity and grace one's passing. Jeanine Awad Shahin (Mama), thank you for being my rock and first example of beauty and grace. Love and gratitude to my sister, Michele, and my brothers, Charles and John, and your beautiful families. To the Naif Shahin, Abraham Shaheen, and Khalil Awad families: I am blessed to come from you. To the Margaret Hoatland and James E. Wood family: I am honored to be part of your clan. To my siblings-in-law, Emily, Albert, and Jimmy, and your beautiful families, thank you.

INFLUENCES

Jesus, Mother Mary, Khalil Gibran, Beatles, John Lennon and Yoko Ono, G. I. Gurdjieff, Maxwell Maltz, Ralph Nader, Shirley Chisholm, Jethro Kloss, Todd Rundgren, Christiane Northrup, Suzanne Arms, Deepak Chopra, Mary Beth Janssen, and Dr. Joe Dispenza

HERBAL PRACTITIONERS

Kate Gilday, Jean Argus, Pam McNew, and Lisa Fazio

ENERGETIC PRACTITIONERS

Carol Fitzpatrick and Mark Torgeson, Susan Beadle, Susan Roback, Lena Moon, Betty Ann Petkovsek, Lisa Monohan, Kimberly Farrell, and Caren Direen

ORGANIZATIONS

Kids Against Pollution (KAP), New York Public Interest Research Group, New York State Labor & Environment Network, Citizen's Environmental Coalition, Healthy and Clean New York, National Council of Churches Eco-Justice Working Group, Antiochian Orthodox Archdiocese of North America, Global Warming Action Network (GWAN)

HENNA EXPERTS

Catherine Cartwright-Jones (The Henna Page and Henna for Hair), Heather Caunt-Nulton (Artistic Adornment), Neeta Desai Sharma, and Julie Trainer

There is a prevailing illusion that our success comes from our sole efforts, when in truth there is no success without those who wish us well and hold space for our success.

Beautiful Sister Blasé Sylvester, thank you for being a beauty cohort and for showing me that I AM a success story as-is.

To Wendy Meyerson, thank you for giving me a chance and for our growth together from employer to friend.

To Karen Farrell Langevin, Aubrey Hampton, and Aubrey Organics: thank you for making me part of your amazing "families."

My thanks also to the following:

Teri Dunn Chase, Robyn Miller, Peter Richard, Linda Hennings, Deirdre Turner, Jackie Michel, Bette Mamone, Rajbir Singh Taneja-Husson, Lynne Micheline, Linda Vincent, Jayne Ritz, David and Richard Taylor, Alice Curtis, Kathy and Brian Kissane, Margaret Haughton, Mary Gressler, Dr. Julie Perlanski, Elaine Cobb, Mary Deluca, Patricia McVeigh, Monica Gondara, Barb Albrecht, Nunziata and Dale Gallagher, Tina Kusela, JoAnne Salamone, Al Chase, Chris Casey, Chris Connolly, Chris Smith, Benjamin Smythe, Dr. Richard Smardon (ESF at Syracuse University), John Manning, Howie Hawkins, Nancy Morelle, and Erin Covey Creative

The KAP Kids: Nick Byrne, Jason Babbie, Kathleen Curtis, Barb Mezzanini, Vickie Thompson, Felicia Davis, Illia Kenney, Anthony Dorsey, Andrew Lamphere, Hayley Carpenter, and Shadia Fayne

The Canal Chicks (www.chicksalongthecanal.com): Juli Webster (Chief Chick), Amber Tabangay (Persnickety Chick), Christina Beck-Hoover (Sassy Chick), and Kelly Crane Liddell (Shabby Chick), with love from Cosmic Chick.

The Tentresses: Jennifer Smith, Christine Kearney, Jennifer Kemp Quintana, Pooniel Bumstead, Kathy Sumner, and Lisa Fazio, all of Crystal Valley Red Tent of Central NY

My deepest heart-felt appreciation to all supporters and patrons of Faces of Astarte; without YOU there is no wellness beauty natural salon/spa. Thank you, every beauty, for your willingness to "go natural," for being open enough to consider herbal mud colorants and paying me to experiment on your hair, and for your willingness to jump in the mud with patience and trust in me to get it right.

Deep gratitude for everyone who volunteered her or his head and time to make this book happen. It takes a village to create a book, including those who so graciously modeled for the photographs in this book — all real mudheads! They are Robyn Chance (thank you for your beauty and grace and makeup artistry), Lydia Barnes, Patricia McVeigh, Elaine Hage, Robin Starring, Kelly Crane Liddell, Tristan Dunn, Sue Beadle, Helen Neet, Sarah Green, Dianne Wright, Steven Wood, Juli Webster, Kassandra Harris, Helen Isom, Lisa Monohan, Emily Esty, Alice Curtis, Katrina Cheney, Jennifer Tinker, and John Gardner.

Thank you, Storey Publishing, and Deborah Balmuth, for seeing value in this offering. To my editor, Sarah Guare, thank you for your patience and gentle guidance; you are an angel. To Alethea Morrison, thank you for the beauty and art you have contributed in so many ways. To all the amazing, talented people at Storey, you create an incredible team!

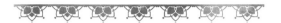

INDEX

Page numbers in *italic* indicate photos; numbers in **bold** indicate charts.

Love your body, love the earth with more Storey books

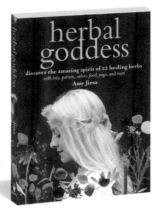

By Amy Jirsa
Boost body, mind, and spirit by working 12 essential herbs into your daily life with this sassy DIY guide.

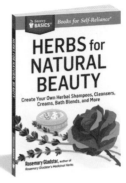

By Rosemary Gladstar
Indulge yourself head to toe with these classic recipes for herbal shampoos and conditioners, massage oils, bath blends, and creams.

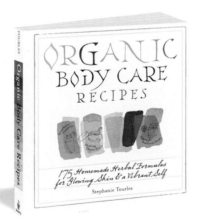

By Stephanie Tourles
Nourish your body while pampering yourself. Whip up all-natural treatments to keep your hair glistening, your face radiant, and your breath fresh.

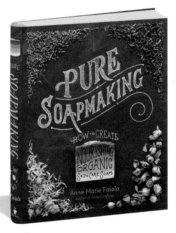

By Anne-Marie Faiola
Wash away the illusion that natural soapmaking is hard with step-by-step photos and recipes for bars laced with everything from almond milk confetti to dandelion zebra stripes.

These and other books from Storey Publishing are available wherever quality books are sold or by calling 1-800-441-5700. Visit us at www.storey.com or sign up for our newsletter at www.storey.com/signup.